English Editing: Eliana Carter
Contact: Dr.Arditti1@gmail.com

ISBN 9798865292715

HORMONE HACKING

The Functional Medicine Approach to Treating
Fatigue, Obesity, Hypothyroidism, and More

DR. ALEXANDER ARDITTI

Contents

Please note

Because most people do not know the medical terms that appear in this book, you will get the most benefit from it by referring to the List of Terms that appears at the end of the book. It presents an interpretation of words that you may not be familiar with. I recommended you to read the first four chapter to better understanding of the following chapters

There is no choice. You do not have to go back to school. Simply choose to sit down to study early in the morning; that way, it will be easier for you to implement the recommendations written in the book and maintain your health.

Introduction

I wrote this book to answer the questions many individuals ask me about their problems. I explained to them that it is caused by hormonal dysfunction and hypothyroidism to them and tried to help them understand the problems associated with thyroid disease and how they can be resolved using natural substances. In this book, you will find a detailed explanation of many enzymatic processes that are involved in thyroid function and how the gland produces its hormones. To feel healthy and happy, you need to know what is going on in your body. You cannot function optimally if the body does not have enough energy. Only the body's natural substances can produce energy —not drugs or medications. A similar situation occurs with your car. It is powered by gasoline; if you accidentally put diesel or water in it, of course, it won't be able to take you anywhere. The same thing can be said about drugs. Some people get angry when a particular "life-saving" drug is not added to their "medicine basket." I have proven many times that drugs do not save lives, reduce symptoms (except for antibiotics), or improve the results of laboratory tests. They never heal. If they worked in some situations, often new problems would appear because of them while the old disease continued to cause damage. Sometimes, an entirely new illness will appear.

I tried to write about these processes in as simple a language as possible, but you might need to know some terminology. You need to take a break to take care of your health. Sit down for at least an hour a day—do this early in the morning when no one will disturb you—and write down in a notebook the terms you don't know. I wrote key terms at the end of the book with a short explanation of each. You need to learn these terms to understand what is happening in your body when you do not feel well. There is no choice. I recommended reading the first four chapters first to understand the following chapters. You don't always get answers to your medical problems from the treating doctor and may end up wandering from doctor to doctor with the hope of finding relief. Many years ago, as a young doctor, I consulted my colleagues and did not always find an answer to my medical problems. I had to look for the cause and find new methods of treating my medical issues instead of taking medicine. That's why I left conventional medicine and concentrated on a relatively new branch of internal medicine called *functional medicine*. That way, I have been able to live another 35 years with a good quality of life.

Functional medicine's approach is to restore the body to its normal level of functioning by using the natural substances it produces or by getting them from food. A lack (or excess) of essential biological substances over a long period of time can cause some diseases to develop. With the help of *a new method to interpret laboratory tests accurately and correctly*, you can understand what is going on in your body. If there is a lack (or excess) of biological substances, a specific area in your body or all of your body will not function correctly. Only when you return your body's condition to the way it was when you were young will all your complaints subside and vitality return to you. I wrote this book because I was already near death, but I wanted to live. In this book, I discuss widespread symptoms that conventional medicine does not treat correctly: fatigue, hypothyroidism problems, menstrual disorders, infertility, epilepsy, psychiatric disorders, and fibromyalgia. I recently added attention-deficit/ hyperactivity disorder (ADHD) to the list of problems that may respond to my therapeutic approach. One of my own children and myself suffered from this disorder, but I managed to improve without medication.

I recently added a chapter on ADHD in adults—you might recognize yourself or your friends in this chapter. Because the topics in this book are probably unfamiliar to you, and because many people do not understand the terms used in this book, you should know that it takes time to learn the terminology. Therefore, I offer you another way to learn. If you suffer from one of the diseases mentioned in this book, talk to your doctor about the issue; your doctor may be interested in learning something new. If not, look for a doctor who practices alternative medicine within the framework of your healthcare system. If a doctor shows interest, print the chapter and give it to him or her this book as a gift. It might get thrown in the trash. But if you're lucky, your doctor will read it and do his or her best to help you after learning more and getting a new perspective on your illness.

During your lifetime, you will see changes in body functions resulting from life itself and from stress, sensitivity to different food or environmental substances or medications, or to meals containing many chemicals and other unnatural substances. It will be possible for me to add new topics to this book in the future that readers come up with to clarify a particular issue or answer an essential query a second time. So I hope the book never gets old.

I am Spanish in origin; I was born in Uruguay and have had the Family Name Caballero on my mother's side of the family since my family's expulsion from Spain in the 15th century. Today I am 85 years old and happy to be able to continue answering your questions about my good life in the time I have to do so. Send your comments to Dr.Arditti1@gmail.com. I will only answer questions about topics related to the book, however. With a little effort, you will find answers to your questions in this book. I was happy to help many patients using their body's natural substances for many years. Most of their complaints were related to underactivity of the thyroid gland, particularly in women who were trying to cope with irregular periods, difficulty getting pregnant, and symptoms of allergies. At the root of all of these issues may lie a single problem: a lack of cellular energy. When these complaints are not handled correctly, the result is a decrease in quality of life over many years, as well as personal problems. I think women deserve an excellent quality of life and a healthy body and mind, because we only live once. Of course, men need to take care of themselves, too!

Chapter 1

The Spring of Life Is Founded in Mitochondrial Health!

You must have noticed that a child can appear to run non-stop, and sometimes adults have difficulty catching up with them. By contrast, an older adult should move more carefully and use a cane or a walker to keep from falling. What is the reason why a young person looks more energetic than an older adult? A young person produces a tremendous amount of energy particles to activate the body. This energy is necessary for the body. It's like fuel for a car: The more power a person produces, the better the chance of winning world records in sports.

An adult, however, does not produce enough energy particles to activate his muscles, brain, or body. Something changes over the years. The adult becomes weaker and subject to disease because of a lack of energy to activate the enzymatic systems that are necessary to propel the body and prevent disease. Sometimes I see a young person producing sufficient power but experiencing blockage of this energy in some areas of the body where energy particles do not enter the cells sufficiently. A blockage in one of the stations in the body where energy is created or where hormones that produce energy enter the cell is a widespread phenomenon, and removal of these barriers is required for good health.

One living wonder is that animals, plants, and humans can produce energy particles by themselves. This phenomenon raises at least two questions: (1) How is this energy made in our body; and (2) how can a human being use this energy and maintain it throughout life?

During the 13th century, many expeditions were launched to search (without success) for the source of life (Figure 1-1). Still, during life, we lose our ability to produce this energy. In the modern era, many researchers investigating the laws of natural science and the life sciences have offered answers to these two questions. The answer to the first question is as follows: Energy particles are produced in tiny organelles inside the cells. These organelles were given the name *mitochondria*.

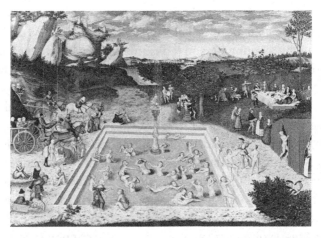

Figure. 1-1. The Fountain of Youth, a 1546 painting by Lucas Cranach the Elder, in Costa Rica. This beautiful place was later destroyed by an earthquake, but it was recently reconstructed.

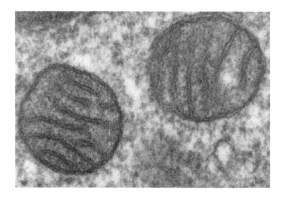

Figure 1-2. View of two mitochondria through an electron microscope. Although usually oblong in shape, like a cigar, they can also appear round when they are cut transversely. Their ability to change shape allows them to get close to areas of the cell in need of energy.

Mitochondrion

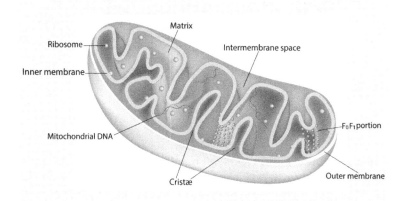

Figure 1-3. The mitochondrion contains a folded inner membrane with an enzyme system to produce energy. Between the folds lies the matrix, which contains enzymes that break the food down into two particles: NAD+ & NADH+ The enzyme system in the inner membrane transfers electrons from one enzyme to the next. With oxygen, it finally produces ATP particles, which contain a high level of energy that is distributed freely into the cells.

Millions of years ago, during the development of life on Earth, a bacterium entered the first cell that was created and produced energy particles, as all bacteria do. This allowed the cell to divide (thereby reproducing) and produce the energy necessary to build tissues and create new life. A single cell can contain as many as 100 (even more) of these "invasive" bacteria, which became known as *mitochondria* (Figures 1-2 & 1-3). These organelles provide the energy required to activate the many components of the cell, especially its enzymatic systems (Figure 1-3). They can maintain the normal metabolism in the body. *Metabolism* is the term used to describe all the chemical reactions that occur in the body.

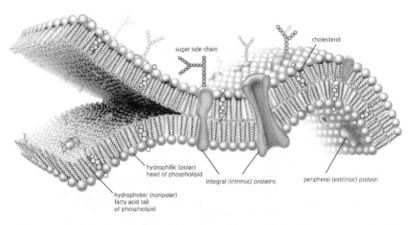

Figure 1-5. Structure of a typical cell membrane. Note the arrangement of the two layers of cholesterol making the membrane permeable and which has receptors that permit the controlled entrée of specific substances like hormones into the cell

I admire the body's ability to produce its own energy particles to activate itself. Energy stores are usually used to power your car or the appliances in your home. However, every living thing produces energy as needed—even plants. Often the process involved in producing energy is related to human health, because without the cell's ability to produce energy, the body might develop many diseases, including high cholesterol, high blood glucose, obesity, brain disorders, muscle weakness, and liver dysfunction. Thus, if the mitochondria in our cells do not produce enough energy, they change their shape (Figures 1-6), the brain will not function well, the heart muscle will not contract efficiently, and the liver will not turn certain substances and hormones into active substances or neutralize toxins, because the enzymes that help perform that work do not receive enough energy particles to function within the cells.

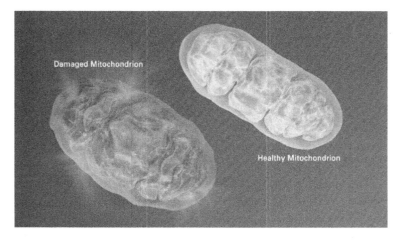

Figure 1-6. A damaged mitochondrion.

In my opinion, mitochondria are the source and fountain of life for all of us because of their role in the creation of life on earth. The body only needs appropriate food (fuel) for an independent source of energy to function and live. This process is carried out further through the mitochondria, which can finish the final process of breaking down every component of the food that we eat. We are lucky to live in these times, we don't need to travel far because everything that our bodies need to be healthy is right at our fingertips. You only have to know what the body needs. From food, the mitochondria produce two important essential substances: an enzyme called NAD+ (nicotinamide adenine dinucleotide) and NADH+. The short video explains how mitochondria produce energy particles called ATPs. Note the presence of coenzyme Q10 in the mitochondrion's inner membrane. Along with oxygen, mitochondria use the breakdown products of sugar, proteins, and fats to create ATPs and emit carbon dioxide, water, and free radicals—just as your car emits the end products of the fuel it uses for energy. We must maintain the production of these two enzymes throughout life. Both NAD+ and NADH+. They are necessary to activate a large group of enzymes that deactivate genes associated with aging, as well as enzymatic systems that are active during the day and others that are active at night. As you will read later, this explains the origin of some diseases. Sleep disorders, a lack of oxygen, overeating of carbohydrates or proteins, and physical inactivity are the bases of many chronic diseases. People who do not know and follow nature's laws are at risk of developing many diseases.

The energy particles called ATPs decrease in number over the years as a result of damage to mitochondrial enzyme systems or a lack of the vitamins, hormones, and minerals necessary for their activity. These deficiencies result in a reduction in NAD+ levels. Low NAD+ levels have been found in people with many diseases, such as diabetes, obesity, various inflammatory diseases, obesity, and fatigue. Therefore, we need to pay attention to the laws of nature and act accordingly. I will indicate what we need to do and everything required to maintain a normal relationship between these two groups of enzymes. You cannot check the NAD+ levels in your cells using standard laboratory tests. Instead, I assume that some organ in your body is not functioning correctly measuring your body temperature, decoding your blood test correctly and identifying it according to your complaints.

The *answer to the second question is as follows*: Given that the mitochondria function as sources of energy that is essential for life, what can you do to keep them active for most of your life and, thus, prevent diseases as much as possible? The answer to this question is a bit more complex than the answer to the first, because you need to know about several things before you can answer it:

1. The mitochondria have their own DNA, which you inherit from your mother. You inherit the nuclear DNA from your father.
2. The enzymatic systems in the body have a short lifespan and constantly need to be refreshed.
3. You need to know what substances the mitochondria need to function.
4. You need to know what foods you should eat.
5. You need to know what substances inside or outside the body can interfere with mitochondrial activity.
6. Mitochondria produce waste particles called free radicals. These are substances with an uncoupled electron. Thus they are electrically unstable and tend to join with any other substances. Then, these products can alter the molecular structure of lipids, proteins, and DNA, thereby triggering various human diseases. They can influence the enzymatic systems in the body. The active lifetime of biological substances in the body varies greatly—from a few seconds to a week. When their function comes to an end, some vitamins and minerals are activated through a chemical reaction in the liver; alternatively, they can be provided in their active form through food. There are enzymes whose activity is short and constantly needs to be refreshed by the hormones various glands secrete. Each of these hormones has a specific purpose that is determined by a particular gene contained within the DNA of the mitochondria or the cell nucleus. The code for that gene causes it

to duplicate itself, in a way similar to a computer program. You need an adequate amount of hormones in your blood to constantly refresh the enzyme pool in every part of the body. As we will see in the next chapter, glands change the amount of hormones they secrete over a lifetime. Fewer ATPs are produced over time because of our failure to refresh enzymes in the mitochondria and in the cell nucleus. This condition affects the metabolism in the body, which begins to decline.

You also need to know what substances the mitochondria need to function. One factor that can cause mitochondria to reduce their production of energy particles is nutritional deficiency (for example, through the frequent use of digital microwaves to cook or to heat food, which can cause the destruction of vitamins). In addition to hormones, mitochondria and cell enzymes need vitamins and minerals to function well. When there is a deficiency in one or more nutrients, the body reserves them for the vital organs, such as the brain and heart, at the expense of other organs to ensure the body's survival.

In other words, the heart and brain will continue to function at the cost of liver and muscle activity. Therefore, the liver will not be able to neutralize the various toxins that reach it; when this happens, we will not be able to activate our muscles effectively. When our muscles cannot function properly, we complain of fatigue and not being able to use them as we wish.

In general, mitochondria need the following nutrients to work well:

- Minerals: magnesium, calcium, selenium, potassium, zinc, iron, and copper
- Fats: omega 3, olive oil, and cholesterol
- Vitamins: All of the B vitamins, as well as vitamins A, D, E, and K
- Dietary supplements: to maintain a high level of antioxidants, such as carnosine, alpha lipoic acid, coenzyme A100, and N-acetyl cysteine (NAC)

- Hormones: triiodothyronine (T3); insulin-like growth factor-1 (IGF-1), and the sex hormones (estradiol, progesterone, and testosterone).

All of these supplements can be obtained online.

To ensure an adequate supply of NAD+ and NADH+, we need to do the following:
- Prevent nutritional deficiencies
- Exercise every day
- Expose our skin to the sun for at least half an hour a day (without sunscreen)
- Eat natural foods as much as possible.
- Avoid foods containing industrial fats such as canola oil and trans fats
- Sleep at least 8 consecutive hours every night to secrete essential hormones (failure to do so is why people with sleep problems tend to get poor health)
- Take nutritional supplements
- Balance your hormones (see Chapter 5)

Why you have to sleep well

Many genetic mutations are created during the day. It's crucial to get a good, deep, refreshing sleep at night so that the *PARP enzymes* can repair them. When a considerable amount of damage is done to the cell's DNA during the day (that is, when genetic mutations occur), PARP enzymes cause the cell to commit suicide or divide into two healthy cells. Normal immune system activity is also required to repair the damage done by these enzymes. If necessary, take 10 milligrams of melatonin. If you are stressed and can't sleep, first take 750 milligrams of GABA (gamma amino butyric acid).

The supplement NAC and other antioxidants increase the

amount of glutathione and superoxide dismutase (also known as SOD) enzymes in the body. These two critical enzymes immediately neutralize free radicals to prevent tissue damage (this will be discussed later in this book).

The thyroid hormone T3 helps the mitochondria increase the body's metabolic rate by using sugar, cholesterol, and some proteins efficiently to produce the enzyme NAD+. This enzyme is responsible for the adequate functioning of the brain, liver, gastrointestinal system, and heart. These organs require a high level of energy. Low levels of NAD+ have been found in people with various illnesses, including diseases with signs of inflammation. An adequate amount of NAD+ is necessary to improve the response of the immune system in people with autoimmune diseases.

- A low level of NAD+ is associated with the following:
- Aging
- Decreased supply of oxygen to the cells
- Cancer
- Mental fatigue due to chronic fatigue syndrome, fibromyalgia, and autoimmune diseases
- Weight gain
- Depression, Parkinson's disease, and many other mental illnesses
- Cardiovascular diseases
- Diseases associated with mitochondrial dysfunction, including obesity, diabetes, and high cholesterol
- A deficiency in the B vitamins, vitamin D, and others

Here are several ways you can increase your NAD+ level:
- Expose yourself to a cold temperature for 1 to 2 minutes. This can be achieved by sleeping at a room temperature of 19 to 21 degrees Celsius or by dipping your body in cold water for a minute after showering
- Get a half hour of physical activity

- Try intermittent fasting: Have two main meals (one in the morning and one in the afternoon) and either skip dinner or limit it to a small protein-rich meal
- Take Resveratrol (200 milligrams or more)
- Increase your consumption of vitamin E and C-rich fruits or juices in the morning and throughout the day
- Sleep 8 to 9 hours continuously
- Use an AMPK supplement. This supplement (also known as AMP-activated protein kinase) removes waste that has accumulated in your body cells and mitochondria. Using an AMPK supplement is like cleaning the house or using a computer program
- Balance your hormones at the level of someone 20 years of age
- Reduce your stress level and resolve personal conflicts by doing meditation or yoga

Disturbances in sleep and in the night/day cycle, along with stress, are the leading causes of a chronic decrease in NAD+ and an increase in cortisol. Chronic stress turns off the genes that oversee the production of ATP-generated energy in the cell during the night and day. The rise in cortisol at night also explains why failing to get a refreshing sleep stops the production of essential hormones at night. At a specific moment in the body, the metabolic processes are not what nature wanted at that particular time of day or night. The day/night cycle is activated by specific genes, which activate enzymatic systems at one particular time. When this sequence of events goes wrong, the body functions in a different way. As a result, the NAD+ level decreases and diseases such as obesity, diabetes, and many others develop.

To balance the day/night cycle and achieve a deep and continuous sleep, try the following:
- Keep the bedroom completely dark, or wear a blindfold. A

minimal amount of light reaching the eyes results in the cessation of the secretion of melatonin (the "sleep hormone"). Remove the TV screen from the bedroom.

- Increase hormonal secretion at night.
- Avoid large meals before bed; a *small, protein-only* meal—consisting of cottage cheese, fish, tuna, sardines, chicken, red meat, yogurt (with 20 grams of protein), Parmesan cheese, or eggs—*without carbohydrates (including alcohol) is preferred.* During the day, you can include carbohydrates in the main meal in the morning or mid-day. You can also eat a few blocks of chocolate. If you are hungry before you go to bed and eat a large meal with carbohydrates or drink alcohol (that's a carbohydrate, too), you will secrete a lot of insulin and lower your blood sugar level at night. As a result, your body will go into a state of distress and secrete cortisol, or you will wake up in the middle of the night to eat. The nightly secretion of essential hormones (such as thyroid-stimulating hormone [TSH], luteinizing hormone [LH], follicle-stimulating hormone [FSH], and growth hormone [GH]) (Figure 1-4) will stop.

Therefore, the last meal of the day should be light, small, and composed mainly of protein. Thus, you can fast for about 12 to 14 hours until breakfast at 8 am. If you don't take care of your health, the secretion of testosterone decreases, the quality of semen decreases, the menstrual period changes, you stop increasing in height, and you continue to increase in weight and you start to develop a hormonal dysfunction.

Chapter 2

How I Began a Personal Journey With Hormonal Healing

From a young age, I longed to understand how the body works, how blood is produced, how muscles move bones, how our cells work. I suffered from severe asthma, probably on an allergic background. Like a computer engineer learning how the computer works and how to write software—that's how I studied the body. By the age of 27, I had become a doctor. By the age of 60, I had developed many of the diseases that appear at that age. I was working in a high-stress atmosphere and had developed obesity, high blood pressure, and high blood glucose and cholesterol levels. On this health background, I developed a blood cancer called chronic myeloid leukemia, or CML. By accident, I discovered that the levels of essential hormones in my body were deficient. Thus, the body and immune system were weakened, and various diseases had developed that drugs cannot cure. Then a brilliant idea arose in my mind: "I am 60 years old: What would happen if I raised my hormone levels to those of someone aged 20 (which is when I had my best vitality)?" Anyway, I had nothing to lose. I might die with intolerable suffering from acute leukemia, given that at the time (the 2000s), the only treatment available for people with CML was interferon. It was not as easy to get biological hormones then as it is now. To my surprise, all aspects of the disease regressed to normal values, including the number of blood cancer cells. At that time, a new drug for CML appeared: Gleevec. I was fortunate to be included in the study of this drug, and it did its job, curing me definitively of CML. I was happy and healthy again. I decided to leave my senior position at the hospital and leave conventional medicine. I also decided to learn a new professional field—*functional medicine*—and started a private practice in it.

Today, I know that the brain manages all the activity in the body in two ways: voluntarily, as is seen when we activate our muscles to get anywhere; or involuntarily, as is seen when our cells' functions take place under the influence of hormones. The brain controls the trillions of cells in the body through messengers called hormones. They make up the body's operating system. Hormones are the "language" the brain uses to speak to our cells. Those interested in learning this language will maintain a high level of energy for life, an average body weight, a joy of life, and live with fewer diseases, thereby achieving longevity. The hormonal language is the body's way of adapting itself to its constantly changing environment, diets, types and amounts of stress, sleeping habits, and physical activity, as well as to human reproduction. Your diet may change your DNA. The brain's hormones activate glands located in various places in the body and instruct them to secrete their own hormones. As I have learned, energy production decreases from the age of 20 to 60 years as the amounts of hormones secreted by many glands also decrease. I felt very well as I approached my 40s. Without realizing it, however, I was actually getting sick. By the age of 50, I felt unwell because of diabetes, high cholesterol, high blood pressure, significantly excess weight, and cancer.

What would you say if I proved to you that problems such as obesity, fatigue, heart failure, hair loss, depression, heart problems, skin problems, and joint problems are all related to hormonal changes? If you understand the early signs of hormonal decline, you can prevent many diseases before they occur. You might be surprised because you learned something different about your health issues from your doctor. As a conventional doctor, I was also surprised when I discovered that hormones can make the body function efficiently and stay healthy. Since then, my life has changed for the better. I have received tools that allow me to control my body and my life. Doctors don't study the relationship between hormonal decline and disease in university for various obvious reasons. I did not waste time on things that did not contribute to my health or that of my family. Recreation is good from time to time to lower stress. We only live once. If we waste time, we will not have enough time to know why we are sick or how to prevent illness. Conventional medicine does not deal with disease prevention—only with treating people with common diseases using drugs (medication) after the disease appears. Being healthy and functioning correctly at every age or during a late age is your responsibility. It will bring happiness and joy to your family members and, of course, to you. I was motivated to write this book and share my knowledge with you so that you will know what your hormonal situation is and learn how to live with energy, joy, and health while promoting a cure for diseases that may appear at some time during your life. You can do many things by using a hormonal supplement that is adapted to your physiology.

Sometimes you need to consult a doctor who is ready to help you. But with a supportive diet, physical activity, vitamin and mineral supplements, and good sleep, your body will secrete the hormones that you need to stay healthy. You can get your health back and revive the feeling of youth.

Your doctor is only human, however, and faces obstacles to carrying out his or her work. Your doctor may face the decision to prescribe medicines that contain unnatural hormones to prevent depression, for example, or to prevent a woman from becoming pregnant. When you take a small dose of natural or bio-identical hormones (hormones that are 100% identical to those the body produces), you allow your body to function properly and feel good. To help you achieve this, I will use a minor amount of them that have been adjusted precisely to the amount your body created naturally when you were in your 20s or 30s—a time when we feel like we are in heaven. When we are in our 40s or older, the hormonal levels in our bodies are not enough to make us feel that good.

The brain gives instructions through hormones that can activate every gland in the body (Figure 2-1):

- **The hypothalamus**: Also known as the "small brain," the hypothalamus is located in the lower part of the brain. It is connected to every other area of the brain but most directly with the *pituitary gland*, which executes its commands. The hypothalamus is an important brain center, in that it manages everything that happens in the body and reacts to the body's environment. It contains many sensors, which keep track of those aspects of life of which we are not consciously aware, such as the concentration of water in the body, body temperature, hunger, and thirst. It also responds to sensations of rage and aggression. It is an essential intermediary between the nervous system and the pituitary gland, in that it secretes hormones that contain instructions for various glands throughout the body to produce their own hormones. The hypothalamus is like the conductor of an orchestra. In addition to transmitting many instructions to the pituitary gland, it can trigger the production of a specific hormone to maintain the balance among all the hormones in the body in response to various influences originating in the body itself or from external sources.

- **The pituitary gland.** This small, pea-sized gland plays a central role in the ability of the body to maintain its vitality and general well-being. The pituitary gland is called the "father gland," because it uses the instructions it receives from the hypothalamus to control the hormone-secreting activity of most of the other glands in the body. Specifically, this gland secretes adrenocorticotropic hormone (also known as ACTH), thyroid-stimulating hormone (TSH), growth hormone (GH), luteinizing hormone (LH), follicle-stimulating hormone (FSH), and prolactin to instruct other glands to secrete their own hormones.

- **The pineal gland:** The pineal gland, which is in the brain, secretes melatonin (the "sleep hormone") and lets the body know whether it is day or night.

- **The thyroid gland:** The thyroid gland, which is in the neck, produces the hormones inactive thyroxine (T4) and the active triiodothyronine (T3) in response to TSH. These thyroid hormones manage energy and heat production in the body. The thyroid gland also secretes calcitonin and parathyroid hormone, which help maintain the balance between calcium and phosphorus in the body and the balance of these two hormones against other hormones in the body.

- **Liver and kidneys:** The liver and kidneys convert T4 into its active form, T3; growth hormone into its active form, insulin-like growth factor (IGF)-1; and many vitamins into their active forms as well. They also neutralize many toxins before removing them from the body in urine or feces.

- **Adrenal glands:** The adrenal glands, which lie just above the kidneys, secrete four essential hormones using cholesterol as the raw material: *dehydroepiandrosterone* (also known as DHEA), which serves as raw material for making sex hormones; *cortisol,* which manages the body in stressful situations; *aldosterone,* which controls the water-salt balance in the body; and *pregnenolone,* which controls memory in the brain. Cholesterol is used to produce these hormones.
- **Testicles:** A pair of glands inside the scrotum that produce sperm and male hormones, including testosterone, which supports male fertility. *Testosterone* is an inactive hormone that is converted to its active form—dihydrotestosterone—inside body cells.
- **Ovaries:** A pair of female glands that secrete *estradiol and progesterone* to manage the menstrual cycle and women's fertility.
- **Pancreas:** An organ found in the left abdominal area that secretes *insulin*, which has an effect on blood sugar levels.
- **Thymus:** A gland located in the chest whose role is to maintain normal immune system activity. Its activity is supported by T3, IGF-1, and the sex hormones.

Here's a seven-step guide for optimal health:
1. In the morning, open a window to inform your brain that a new day has arrived. In the morning or during the day, go outside to expose parts of your skin to the sun's rays for half an hour. This will help your pineal gland secrete melatonin the following night to help you sleep.
2. Go to bed at the same time every day (for example, between 9 pm and 10 pm) and get up at the same time (6 am-7 am) each morning.
3. Reduce stress to prevent a buildup of cortisol, which disrupts

the day/night cycle and has a negative effect on the secretion of the sex hormones, thyroid gland, and melatonin at night.

4. Exercise for a half hour at regular times—preferably between 5:00 pm and 6:00 pm in the evening, when your cortisol level is low. This physiological state allows a significant amount of growth hormone and testosterone to be secreted during training, especially when you take 50 grams of protein powder before and after the workout If you eat a small protein-rich dinner, you will continue to secrete essential hormones at night because you will be able to sleep deeply. You will also develop a large muscle mass as the amount of orexin your body produces increases. *Orexin* is an enzyme that transports chemicals produced by specialized brain cells between nerve cells in the brain. It allows us to maintain alertness and lean body weight by burning calories and balancing our blood sugar levels against the functional needs of the internal organs. A lack of orexin is one of the mechanisms involved in reducing the number of calories burned. People who gain weight then become depressed.

5. Avoid activities that reduce orexin levels, including a high-carbohydrate diet, increased sugar consumption (which makes you feel tired and sleepy), untreated inflammatory conditions, food allergies, and lack of sleep.

6. To prevent a decrease in NAD+, resolve inflammatory conditions caused by viruses, bacteria, or autoimmune diseases. These conditions sharply increase the concentration of free radicals, which can damage body tissues and mitochondria. An excess of free radicals can be reduced by increasing your intake of antioxidants from foods or nutritional supplements—such as N-acetyl cysteine (NAC), which increases glutathione and SOD enzymes to neutralize free radicals immediately.

7. Follow a diet consisting of natural foods that include meat, fish, vegetables, and dietary fiber. Avoid processed foods,

smoked food, deep-fried foods, or foods that have undergone industrial processing through the addition of chemicals and unsaturated fats. Polyunsaturated fats (PUFAs) may block hormone receptors on the surface of cells, thereby blocking the entry of hormones into the cells (I will explain this later).

Consider this: Milk and milk products contain 0.5 grams to 0.8 grams of unsaturated fat for every 100 grams. [Personally, I minimize this amount by using organic milk and milk products.] By including milk and milk products in your diet, you can easily consume 5 to 10 grams or more of unsaturated fat (PUFA's) per day. A diet high in fats or sugar disrupts the day/night cycle and reduces NAD+ levels in the blood. Processed foods overwork the liver by presenting it with many chemicals that have to be neutralized and decrease the rate of conversion of T4 to its active form, T3. We live in very toxic environments, with toxins found in food, the air, and water. We need to allow our liver to do its job effectively to neutralize all of these toxic factors. To do so:

1. Eat many colorful fruits such as blueberries, dark grapes, and strawberries.
2. Don't eat too many simple carbohydrates, because they will disturb your sleep and the day/night cycle of enzymatic activity, which can result in a fatty liver, liver dysfunction, decreased thyroid gland activity, and a deficit of energy.
3. Choose your meat carefully. Many meats, such as chicken and beef, become contaminated when cattle ranchers use feeds containing industrial fats. To avoid this, you may need to buy meat from a place where they raise free-range cattle and organic poultry.
4. Avoid eating too many carbohydrates or drinking alcohol just before going to bed. The hormones necessary for our regular development are secreted during the first hours of deep sleep,

and a bedtime intake of carbohydrates and alcohol can interfere with this natural process.

In conclusion: If you want to avoid diseases as much as possible and enjoy a good quality of life, especially in your old age, you need to maintain the continuous activity of the mitochondria and avoid any factor that can interfere with its function.

Endocrine system mele-female

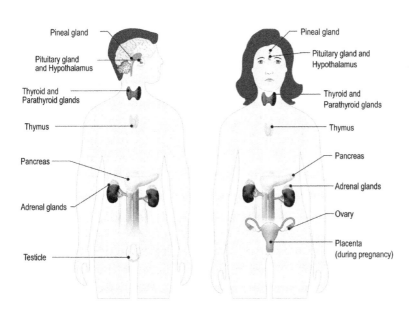

Figure 2-1: The primary hormonal system in humans. The glands in the brain respond to information they receive from within the body and from its environment. They help in the production and secretion of hormones, which carry chemical messages to every cell in the body to motivate the body to maintain its hormonal balance at each and every moment. This allows us to develop and adapt to our environment after hormones affect the activity of genes.

The Hippocampus

The hippocampus is the memory center of the brain. It stores information about all of the events that occur in our lives through all of our senses, which makes it similar to a super-computer. The hippocampus is constantly listening, picking up signals from the many types of atoms that are uniquely arranged in our body and in everything else on earth and re-cording these signals for future reference. For example, if you eat bread that does not contain gluten, the hypothalamus will record the atomic composition of bread as "gluten-free" in its memory the first time this bread is encountered. The second time you eat bread, but it contains gluten, the memory center will inform you of a change in the atomic composition of the bread and transmit instructions to other parts of the brain to trigger contraction of the intestinal muscles (resulting in diar-rhea and vomiting) or respiratory tract (resulting in an asthma attack) as a warning. If we continue to eat bread with gluten, a disease may develop. The same happens when the body is in contact with a "real" foreign substance. Given that we live in very toxic environments, knowing that the hippocampus can warn us about the entrance of foreign entities into our bodies can be comforting. These warnings can be avoided, of course, by limiting your meals to the natural foods you ate the first time (But you may also have an allergic reaction to natural foods—vitamin C, eggs, milk etc. —because they change its molecular structure during the time). When we take drugs, the hippocampus may inform us that the body has not accept-ed their composition. The result is a reaction categorized as a "side effect." Animals have a highly developed hypothalamus and teach small animals what to eat. We inherited that from the prehistoric man (Figure 2-2).

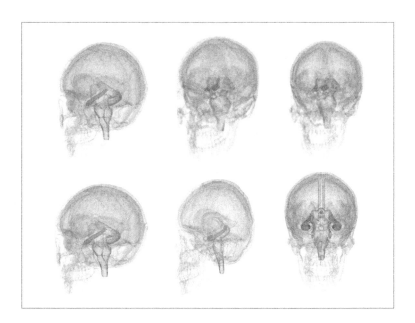

Figure 2-2 . Six views of the hippocampus.
(Taken from en-wiki: File_Hippocampus.htm)

Hormonal symphony

Each hormone has a special and unique role in the body. All the hormones in the body work together, however, influencing each other and cooperating with each other to permit all aspects of the body to work together in harmony. This is similar to an orchestra that plays a particular symphony under the baton of the central conductor's hypothalamus. Each instrument has the notes to play and knows the rhythm to keep. Still, they are all required to play a complete and harmonious piece. For example, testosterone increases the secretion of the hormone IGF-1 and vice versa.

At the same time, without a suitable and balanced diet, the body will not be able to produce the variety of hormones it needs in the quantities needed. Hormones bind to genes in the

DNA of the cell and reproduce their instructions, usually by instructing the DNA to make copies of specific enzymes or other substances found in the cell. You first must provide the body with an appropriate quantity and quality of raw materials. The body is composed of proteins, saturated fats, and water. It produces its hormones and enzymes from amino acids, which make up proteins, or from cholesterol. Much of the food in the modern diet is so highly processed and industrialized that you can easily find yourself with a hormonal problem, even if you consider your diet to be healthy. Your diet must provide the raw materials needed to support the hormonal system (and not interfere with it). Sometimes laboratory tests reveal a low and insufficient level of a specific biological substance; we then take supplements to support its function. An experienced naturopath can offer you a delicious diet rich in essential food components, with surprising adjustments to avoid or treat various hormonal problems.

It would be best, however, if you remembered that no matter how healthy your diet is or how much physical activity you perform, at a certain point in life and for various reasons, your body will produce less and less of all its hormones (Figures 2-3 to 2-6). This usually occurs after you reach your 40s—sometimes at an earlier age, depending on your lifestyle and diet. The decline in hormonal secretions leads to a gradual decrease in physical function. You will complain about a symptom that was not there before. You will go to the attending physician and receive some medicine designed to reduce your complaints and improve the results of your laboratory tests, or you may be put through a series of tests to find the cause of your complaints. If all of the test results are "normal," there is likely a hidden hormonal imbalance. This is because practitioners of conventional medicine usually do not test the entire hormonal system. Even if they do, they will interpret the results as being "within normal limits." In the end, many patients continue to complain and look for therapeutic methods to resolve these complaints. When a hormonal problem is discovered, doctors usually only address that single hormone and ignore all the others that need to be in balance with it to maintain the body's normal function.

For example, when they discover a problem with the thyroid gland, they prescribe the natural T4 hormone, which is identical to the hormone produced in the thyroid gland. They ignore the fact that this gland does not work alone; rather, it is part of a system of hormones, all of which need to be in balance with each other. The thyroid gland may slow down the activity of other glands for many reasons. It may result, for example, in excess estradiol (the female sex hormone) or excess cortisol (the stress hormone). Thus, it is essential to treat all hormones and not just one. It's like a problem on the city roads. The mayor may only take care of a single road, but you know other roads must be addressed—just as you understand that other hormones are probably involved if one hormone is out of balance.

The problem with the hormonal treatment given today is that conventional medicine uses drugs that contain hormones that are not biological, meaning they are different from the hormones the body produces and their blood levels do not show up in the results of blood tests. A single hormone is often given in huge quantities, rather than the entire system. This brings temporary relief but sometimes worsens the problem; at the very least, it does not help the patient in the long run. Many people still suffer from symptoms of hormonal hypoactivity and look for a solution from another pharmaceutical company from India!, despite the fact that the other companies produce a table that contains the same natural T4 hormone. Biologicals have no side effects because natural hormones are used by the body's cells. The cause of hormonal hypoactivity may not be a lack of T4 but, rather, the hormone is blocked and cannot enter the cells or fail to convert T4 (an inactive hormone) into T3 (an active hormone), as you will learn later. Over time, a lack of proper hormone treatment may cause the patient's health to worsen as all of the hormonal systems go out of balance.

Treatment with natural biological hormones in amounts that are as close as possible to the levels your body would have produced at a young age can make you feel the same health and vitality that you felt back then. I will teach you the method that worked for me and hundreds of others in my clinical practice. You will find that when your hormones are out of balance, you may consider supporting them with a diet and exercise plan. You will still need bioidentical hormones in balance to feel vitality, however.

What are your hormones doing?

The glands in our bodies produce hundreds of hormones and secrete them into the bloodstream at a rate of thousands of billions of units per day. There are also hormones that the cells in the digestive system produce locally to break down the food we eat and help the body absorb vitamins and minerals from this food. Hormones can produce energy and heat. They regulate the heart rate and breathing; they make a woman and a man fertile. They help you fall asleep at night and wake you up in the morning.

The hormones may also determine your:
- Blood pressure
- Bone strength
- Muscle tone
- Rate of growth (height)
- Rate of burning fat
- Menstrual cycle (for women)
- Fertility
- Blood sugar and cholesterol levels

- Salt and other mineral levels in your blood and tissues
- Immune system activity
- Success with childbirth

Hormones may also help determine your ability to:
- Get pregnant
- Fight stress and fatigue
- Overcome anxiety
- Prevent depression
- Remember things
- Fight allergic reactions
- Reduce inflammation in your body
- Relieve body pain
- Control sexual urges and achieve sexual satisfaction (through oxytocin—the "love hormone")
- Think clearly

It would not be an exaggeration to say that hormones are essential for all the processes that occur in the body, from the smallest to the largest. It is impossible to live without them.

But in our modern environment, or because we are getting older, it is becoming rare to see someone whose average hormonal level remains the same throughout life as it was at a young age. So it turns out you may not enjoy optimal health before and after your 40s. That may mean you're dealing with fatigue, stress, heart disease, hair loss, obesity, a decreased sex drive, or joint problems—these are all signs of a long-term drop in hormone levels. Medication can only reduce your complaints, but the cause of your complaints will remain. The plan I offer in this book is designed to help you understand the hormonal language when you feel something is wrong and follow its instructions for your diet, lifestyle, exercise, and sleep so that you can live long and maintain optimal health.

The main activity of the essential hormones

T4 and T3 are secreted by the *thyroid gland*. These two hormones produce energy and heat to stimulate the enzymes that are responsible for the body's metabolism. Thus, they help control your body weight and speed up the rate of blood flow to cause more nutrients, water, oxygen, and other hormones to reach your body organs. T3 and T4 help make your skin soft, supple, and warm, all of which happens thanks to a good blood supply and improved secretion from the sweat glands. These two hormones also keep the muscles and joints flexible and pain-free; prevent your hair from becoming dry or falling out; and prevent water retention and facial swelling; as well as dry skin and various skin diseases, and problems with memory and concentration. They are essential to look young and feel energetic and healthy. The amount of these two hormones decreases over time, however (Figures 2-3 and 2-4). We'll expand on the functions of the hormones secreted by the thyroid gland in the following chapters.

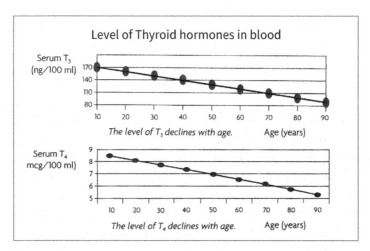

Figure 2-3. Rate of secretion of the main thyroid hormones decreases with age. Top: Rate of change in T3 levels. Bottom: Rate of change in T4 levels. (Taken from T. Hertoghe. Hormonal solution book)

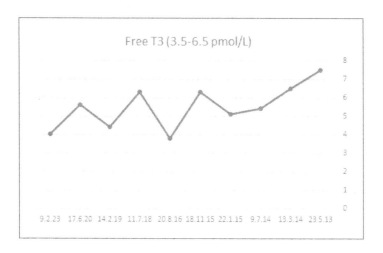

Free T3 (3.5-6.5 pmol/L)

9.2.23 17.6.20 14.2.19 11.7.18 20.8.16 18.11.15 22.1.15 9.7.14 13.3.14 23.5.13

Figure 2-4. My T3 blood levels over a 10-year period. Last year, I used only the active T3 hormone and managed my dose according to body temperature.

Testosterone is essential for women as well as men, although in smaller amounts. It is responsible for sexual satisfaction in both sexes. Figure 2-5 shows the simultaneous decline in sex hormone levels beginning at approximately age 25 years.

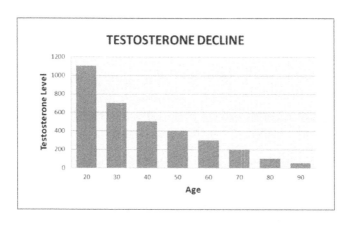

Figure 2-5. Decrease in testosterone over the lifespan (males).

43

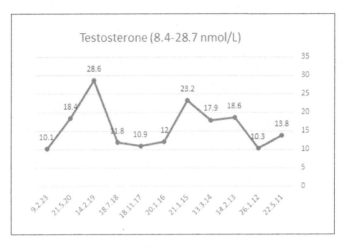

Figure 2-6. My testosterone blood levels over a 10-year period.

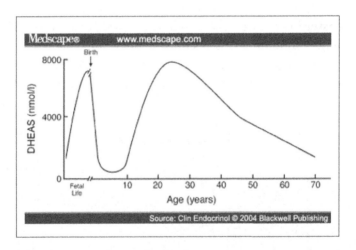

Figure 2-7. A large amount of DHEA is secreted by the adrenal glands in the fetus. It is necessary for normal brain development. The fetus also receives DHEA from its mother. When fetal DHEA levels are low, various neurological disorders can develop. This hormone is essential during the body's development. Note that DHEA level rise again during the school and the university years to be used to produce the sex hormones.

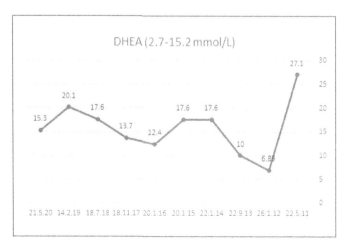

Figure 2-8. My DHEA blood levels over an 8-year period during which I used natural hormones.

Insulin is secreted by the **pancreas** to regulate blood sugar levels. Insulin levels increase with age after age 40 years.

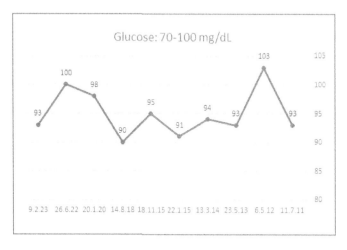

Figure 2-9. My glucose levels over several years after treatment with natural hormones.

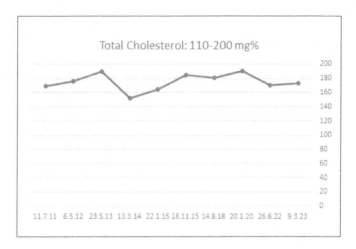

Total Cholesterol: 110-200 mg%

200
180
160
140
120
100
80
60
40
20
0

11.7.11 6.5.12 23.5.13 13.3.14 22.1.15 18.11.15 14.8.18 20.1.20 26.6.22 9.3.23

Figure 2-10. My cholesterol level over several years after treatment with natural hormones.

Estradiol and **progesterone** are secreted by the ovaries to manage the menstrual cycle. They are also found in men but in smaller amounts. In women, estradiol and progesterone decrease in blood levels between the ages of 40 and 50 (Figure 2-10).

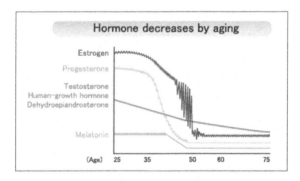

Figure 2-10. Change in the amount of various hormones over the adult lifespan: Everyone experiences a hormonal decline with advancing age. The graph shows the drop in estrogen, testosterone, progesterone, DHEA, and melatonin levels that occurs around the age of 40.

Cortisol is secreted by the adrenal glands. This hormone is called the "stress hormone," because it is secreted in increasing amounts throughout life in response to the development of physiological stress.

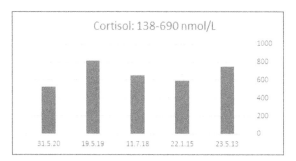

Figure 2-11. My cortisol level during the last 7 years. Like many other physicians, I was under a tremendous amount of stress.

Growth hormone (GH) is necessary throughout life, not just during puberty. Growth hormone is actually a pro-hormone. It is transformed into an active hormone in the liver, where it is converted into its active form, IGF-1 (Figures 2-12 and 2-13). With good levels of IGF-1, you look younger than your age and have much fewer health problems. It is secreted at night according to the special conditions described before, and its level in blood decreases gradually over the remaining lifespan.

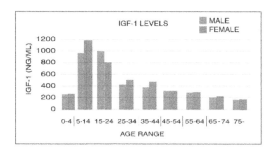

Figure 2-12. Natural IGF-1 hormone levels decrease over time.

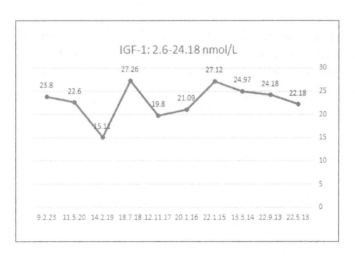

Figure 2-13. My growth hormone output over 10 years with a protein meal before bed. It never goes down.

Melatonin is the sleep hormone. Its primary role is to make you fall asleep at night, secrete nocturnal hormones, and wake up in the morning (Figure 2-14).

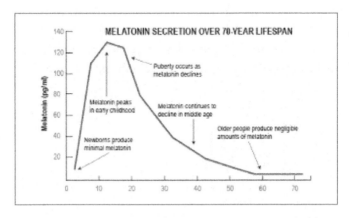

Figure 2-14. Changes in melatonin levels in the blood over the lifespan. Taken from https://www.askdrray.com/tag/melatonin/

Pregnenolone is known as the "memory hormone." It is secreted by the adrenal glands. At a young age, its concentration in the brain is 75 times higher than in the blood. The amount in the brain decreases with age, however, which results in memory disorders (Figure 2-15).

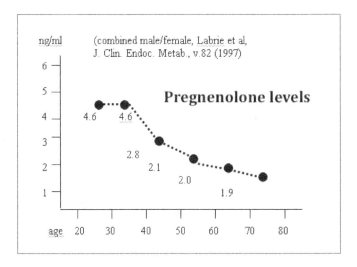

Figure 2-15. Change in pregnenolone levels over the lifespan. Pregnenolone levels start to decrease after about age 30.

Chapter 3

A Huge Biological Role
for the Thyroid Gland

To understand the hormonal activity of the thyroid gland, you need to know how its essential hormones are created. Their activity actually begins in the hypothalamus and ends inside the target cell. The hypothalamus contains a group of cells that function as thermostats, in that they are sensitive to body heat as well as triiodothyronine (T3) levels in the blood.

Thyroid hormone secretion begins when the hypothalamus instructs the pituitary gland to secrete thyroid-stimulating hormone, or TSH. Under the influence of TSH, the thyroid gland releases two hormones into the bloodstream: thyroxine—called T4 for short—which is nearly inactive, and triiodothyronine—called T3 for short—which is the active hormone. T4 bonds with a specific carrier protein that transports it to the liver and kidneys, where it is stored for future use. In these tissues, an enzyme known as 5'deiodinase—called 5'D for short—continuously converts T4 into the active hormone, T3. T3 is secreted from the liver and kidneys into the blood and joins a protein that can carry it to every cell in the body. T3 connected to its T3 receptor in the outer membrane to enter the cell and the mitochondria in each cell and alter the T3 receptor of the mitochondrial membrane, where it is responsible for generating energy; it also enters the cell nucleus, where it interacts with genes that produce chemical reactions that generate heat, raising the body temperature to 37 degrees Celsius (98.6 degrees Fahrenheit) (see Chapter 1).

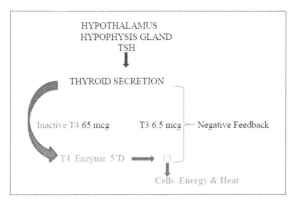

Figure 3-1. Regulation of thyroid hormone secretions

Hormonal equilibrium

The lab blood test in the morning shows the TSH that is secreted mainly at night. Because TSH triggers the thyroid gland to release T4 into the bloodstream, the *free* T4 (FT4) level in the blood also reflects the amount of this hormone that was produced the night before. The free T3 (FT3) blood test results reflect the conversion of T4 to T3 that occurred as a result of 5'D activity in the kidneys and liver, most of which also took place during the night. These values are likely to decrease during the day. For this reason, the most accurate T3 reading value in the morning should lie in the upper level of the average T3 values close to the maximum (Table 3-1). At that level, T3 will induce the production of enough ATP for you to start your workday and maintain a normal body temperature (37.0 degrees Celsius; 98.6 degrees Fahrenheit). The time of day must also be considered when evaluating T4 levels. In the morning, your T4 value is considered adequate if it lies in the center of the average values range for T4 (Table 3-1). That indicates that the thyroid gland has responded well to stimulation by TSH. If the T4 asterisk is below the center of the T4 averages blood values, it indicates that the thyroid gland is sick and has not responded adequately to TSH, or the TSH levels are low because of stress or an inadequate amount of sleep. The secretion of TSH is stable when the body temperature and T3 level are normal. At night, the body temperature falls to 36.5 degrees Celsius (97.7 degrees Fahrenheit). If the thyroid gland is healthy, relatively few TSH molecules are necessary to activate it. Thus, in the morning, the TSH value may be as low as 2. If the thyroid is sick, the body temperature will decrease and the pituitary gland will increase the TSH level to improve thyroid performance. The asterisk for TSH is above 2, perhaps even higher than that. If the thyroid is sick and not able to secrete enough T4 to maintain the normal body temperature, the T4 asterisk will appear below the center of the normal average range.

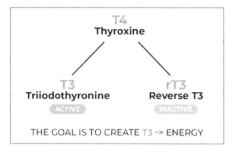

Figure 3-2. The T4/T3 conversion process
Taken from Dr. Momi: instagram.com/functionalthyroidcare

This hormonal equilibrium is maintained through negative feedback. The normal thyroid hormone levels should be as they appear in Table 3-1. The numbers are not important; they will vary among labs because labs use different methods to measure them.

T4/T3 conversion process: a closer look

The job of the enzyme 5'D is to remove one molecule of iodine from T4 (which contains 4 iodine molecules) in the liver and kidneys to transform it into the active hormone T3 and secrete it into the bloodstream. Sometimes 5'D does not work correctly (I will explain why later). For example, it may remove a molecule of iodine from the incorrect position on T4. When this happens, the cell produces another inactive hormone called *reverse T3* (rT3) instead of the normal active T3 (Figure 3-2). The rT3 hormone occupies the receptors on the cell membranes that are usually occupied by T3, thereby blocking its entry into the cell. When T3 cannot enter the cell, it cannot interact with the nucleus or mitochondria in the cell. As a result, the production of body heat and energy shoot downward. Thus, your health depends on the normal activity of this 5'D enzyme. Otherwise, you will find yourself complaining that something is wrong with the way your body is functioning. This event frequently occurs when there is a deficiency in selenium, iron or the hormone progesterone. The body temperature can fall below the range of 36.8 to 37.0 degrees Celsius, which causes the three-dimensional (3D) shape of enzymes to change a little— just enough so they cannot interact with each other. This can cause some enzyme systems to stop functioning normally. If this happens, you start feeling some of the symptoms of inadequate hormonal or mitochondrial activity. The balance between the thyroid hormones is maintained by negative feedback from the active hormone T3 in the blood and the body temperature (Figure 3-1). Normal thyroid hormone levels at all ages must be as shown in Table 3-1.

Table 3-1. Normal thyroid hormone lab test results.

Name	Results	Normal Range
TSH	lower than 2 mIU/L	0.4(.. *.........)4.2
Free T4	15 pmol/L	10(.....*.......)20
Free T3	5.8 pmol/L	3.5(........*....)6.5

Abbreviations: TSH, thyroid stimulating hormone; T4, thyroxine; T3 triiodothyronine.

Suppose it's winter, and the body temperature falls. Immediately, the cells in the hypothalamus start to produce thyroid-releasing hormone (TRH), which transmits chemical instructions to the pituitary gland to secrete TSH. In response to TSH, the thyroid gland immediately starts producing principally its relatively inactive hormone, T4, and its active hormone, T3. It normally secretes 10 times as much T4 as T3 (about 65 micrograms of T4 versus 6.5 micrograms of T3) per day. Other minerals, such as fluorine (the same molecule that is added to drinking water to prevent tooth decay), can compete with iodine for a place in the tyrosine molecule. For this reason, drinking lots of fluoridated water can cause the thyroid gland to become underactive.

Thyroid peroxidase (TPO) is an enzyme that works inside the colloid (a fat-protein medium) in the thyroid gland connecting iodine to the amino acid tyrosine to create T4 and T3. The colloid, which fills cell-bound cavities within the thyroid gland, is called thyroglobulin (TG). Over a 24-hour period, the thyroid gland secretes 80% of its T4 into the blood circulation but only 20% of its T3. The enzymes that release T4 and T3 to the bloodstream need vitamins A, D and C to function optimally. The amount of T3 released into the blood by the thyroid gland is not enough to meet the physiological needs of the body. The rest is gained through the conversion of T4 to T3 outside the thyroid gland (specifically, in the liver and the kidneys).

The lifespan of the T4 hormone is about a week; the lifespan of T3 is only a few hours. T4 is a biologically weak hormone; it produces very little energy or heat. T3 is four times more active than T4. Perhaps for this reason, T4 serves mainly as a pre-hormone, or raw material, for the manufacture of T3. To ensure a sufficient supply of T3 to meet the body's needs, T4 must be constantly converted to T3. Most of this conversion process takes place in the liver and kidneys and is strongly dependent on the "mood" of the enzyme 5'D.

1. As the active thyroid hormone, T3 is responsible for many things that happen in the body. For this reason, there are T3 receptors on the outer surface of every cell and the internal membranes within the cell (on the mitochondria and nucleus), as well. T3 must make a precise connection with its receptor on each membrane to gain entry into these structures. For this to occur, the receptors must not be occupied by any other molecule, particularly rT3. After T3 enters the mitochondrion (see Chapter 1), it helps transform sugar, cholesterol, and some amino acids, along with oxygen, into ATPs (adenosine triphosphate molecules; see Chapter 1). ATP stores energy in the cell, making it available to the cell components to carry out its vital functions. Oxygen is a critical part of this process: If oxygen does not reach the mitochondria in adequate amount, all enzymatic processes come to a halt and we cease to exist. If the number of molecules of T3, IGF-1 (insulin-like growth factor-1), or sex hormones in the mitochondria is too low (as is seen in older people), fewer ATPs will be produced and none of the body cells will function.

2. Once inside the cell, T3 binds to specific genes that cause a

chemical reaction to take place to produce heat. This heat accumulates until the body temperature reaches approximately 37.0 degrees Celsius (98.6 degrees Fahrenheit). This temperature is necessary to maintain the three-dimensional shape of enzymes in the body. The function of proteins—including enzymes—depends critically on the shape of the molecule. By helping it maintain the structure of these enzymes, it helps the cell carry out its vital functions.

3. If the number of molecules of T3 that reach the mitochondria falls too low, fewer ATPs will be produced and none of your body cells will function properly. Thus, even if only part in the body is not functioning well, you can lose your sense of vitality and health throughout your body.

4. The function of the thyroid hormones may be blocked at many "stations"—the hypothalamus, pituitary gland, thyroid gland, the outer and internal (nuclear and mitochondrial) cell membranes, the blood proteins that carry the thyroid hormones, and the liver and kidneys—by the abnormal activity of the enzyme 5'D or a disease involving these organs The correct interpretation of laboratory blood tests and an accurate body temperature reading may allow the clinician to determine where thyroid activity is blocked and reverse it to get the individual back to good health.

The importance of the body temperature during the day

As explained previously, a T3 test taken in the morning will reflect the amount of T4 that was converted to T3 the night before, whereas the T4 reading will only reflect the amount secreted the night before. The level of T3 activity may change at different times of the day. Why? Because the body tissues constantly utilize T3 to create energy and heat to meet the body's needs.

I can use myself as an example, I am now working on this book. After some time, I feel that I am not concentrating fully, and I feel a little tired. My temperature falls from 36.8 to 36.5 degrees today. Receptors on my hypothalamus detect the drop in temperature and send instructions to my thyroid gland to secrete TSH. Meanwhile, I take a break and drink or eat something. After some time has passed, I feel that my brain is able to work again. This could mean several things:

The T3 level in my brain is rising. This suggests that my morning T3 level is adequate for me to work *several hours* in the morning without any disturbance in my activity.

Feeling tired at mid-day is a sign to take a break; your thyroid hormonal system will automatically resume its production of energy and body heat. If not, it may mean that your 5'D enzyme is not working properly or your thyroid gland is "sick." You can't do a blood test every time, but you can measure your temperature to know if there are enough T3 molecules to produce energy and heat *or see your temperature on a digital thermometer to understand what is going on.*

When we pass the age of 50 (or even before), our hormone levels start to fall (see Chapter 2). Any adult with a deficiency in sex hormones, IGF-1, or T3 may experience the effects of inadequate mitochondrial activity. If these levels fall too far, the individual may require a cane, or even a walker, to get around. Anyone with a severe illness or inflammation is likely to be producing very few ATPs and have a low body temperature—just as I explained in the beginning of Chapter 2.

Body heat and its importance in health

Because the T3 hormone is responsible for keeping the body temperature around 37 degrees Celsius and generating energy, we can learn something from this: The body needs to maintain a constant temperature between 36.8 to 37.2 degrees Celsius (98.2

to 98.9 degrees Fahrenheit) during the day to activate all of the enzymatic systems and maintain the internal stability of the body. T3 activates mechanisms that regulate the body's internal temperature in response to environmental influences, physical activity, sweating, nutrition, digestion, learning, and more. A temperature of 37 degrees allows maximum movement of the body; below 36.8 degrees, enzyme activity slows down (Figure 3-3). We all know how it feels when the body temperature rises above 37 degrees Celsius. You get headaches, you feel fatigued, your appetite decreases, your muscles may ache, and you may feel like you have the flu. This occurs because when the body temperature rises, your metabolic rate changes as the toxins secreted by bacteria and viruses in your body activate genes that not only raise the body temperature, but also create a hostile environment for those microorganisms and alert the immune system to act against them. But what happens when the body temperature drops *below* 37 degrees Celsius? Does this have an effect that we are not familiar with? The answer is yes. When the body temperature drops below 36.8 degrees Celsius (98.2 degrees Fahrenheit), metabolic activity decreases because of a change in the three-dimensional structure of enzymes (enzymes are proteins, the functions of which depend on their three-dimensional structure).

One of the functions of T3 is to maintain an average temperature in the body during the day. Several American doctors use body temperature to evaluate T3 activity. In my opinion, body temperature can help doctors understand the cause of a patient's complaints: there are not enough T3 molecules inside the cells! If the body temperature is lower than 36.8 degrees Celsius (98.2 degrees Fahrenheit), a T3 test will show that it is not in the upper third of normal values: that is, not enough T3 molecules have entered the cells to produce heat and energy!

Those who do not measure their body temperature regularly

do not know about this phenomenon. When I feel tired, my temperature is lower than 36.8 degrees. Let's talk about how thyroid hormones affect body temperature and metabolism. From personal experience, unfortunately, I know that doctors do not treat anyone whose body temperature is lower than 37 degrees, or even 36.2. degrees.

Body temperature and the T3 hormone

Body temperature changes during the day depending on your activity. During physical activity, the temperature rises because the conversion of T4 to T3 is adequate for the cell to provide energy to the muscles. Testosterone and IGF-1 are also released. At night, your body temperature drops by 0.05 degrees to 36.5 degrees Celsius or less (32 degrees Fahrenheit), because another type of 5'D enzyme that is active at night prevents T3 from entering the cell and then you can sleep.

Could there be a situation in which the concentration of T3 inside the cells change, and T3 will not be able to enter the cell or act on it for some reason? Yes, there is such a situation, and from personal experience, I can tell you this happens many times. It occurs when (1) the patient receives a high dose of T4, which turns into rT3, which blocks T3 receptors on cell membrane; or (2) you cook with liquid oils, such as canola oil, or eat foods containing unsaturated oil (such fast foods), which reduces the T4/T3 conversion rate and competes with T3 for entry into the cell.

How can we know if there is enough T3 inside the cells? We cannot measure hormone levels inside the cell, but if the patient complains about being fatigued or he wants to sleep all the time and has a body temperature is lower than 36.8 degrees by mid-day or afternoon, there probably is not enough T3 in the patient's cells.

Is there a way to know if the T4/T3 conversion rate in the

liver and kidneys is OK? The answer is yes: If the T3 level in the blood is in the upper third of the normal range. If the T3 level is in the middle range, the body temperature could be as low as 36.5 degrees or even lower. If the T3 level is in the lower third of the normal range, the body temperature should be about 36.2 degrees or 36.3 degrees Celsius. This is seen during the summer, when air-conditioners are fully activated in emergency rooms or in wards for older people who are waiting for the doctor.

Thus, there is a way to know if the number of active hormones particles in the cells is enough. It involves a simple test that every one of you can do right now at your home.

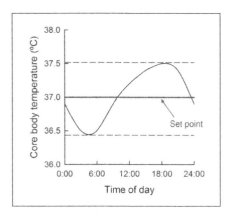

Figure 3-4. The normal body temperature curve over 24 hours. Nighttime temperatures can drop to 36.3 degrees Celsius (97.3 degrees Fahrenheit) by 6 am. During this time, night hormones are being secreted. The body temperature start to rise after the 5'D converters T4 to T3 during the early morning.

Body temperature reflects the activity of the T3 hormone inside the cells. If the body temperature is around 36.8 degrees, T3 molecules should be able to enter the cells in large enough quantities to produce heat and energy sufficiently, and there should be enough T3 into the cells to produce energy. To investigate this possibility, we measure the patient's temperature by placing the thermometer under the patient's tongue and compare it with the normal temperature described in Figure 3-4. Doctors do not consider this simple procedure important;

they will even tell you that your body temperature normally decreases with age. Body temperature does decrease over the years, together with a decrease in mitochondrial activity. So they are right, of course, but they are not taught why. Body temperature is measured using a digital (or other) thermometer placed under the tongue in adults or in young children (in the armpit, you get lower temperature) or in the anus in babies. To perform the test correctly, the thermometer must be held. The temperature is taken after 1 minute of continuous measurement. It is essential to measure the temperature at least twice a day for 3 days. The first measurement should be made in the morning while you are still in bed and recorded on a writing pad placed within easy reach. That temperature should be 36.5 degrees or more. Your body temperature should rise gradually during the morning to about 36.9 or 37 degrees. The second measurement should be made before your mid-day lunch or about an hour after lunch (about 13:00 [1:00 pm]).. After that, it will drop. You will be tired and want to go to sleep because the conversion of T4 to T3 has been stopped by other types of 5'D enzymes.

I take my temperature twice in the morning right after I get up. If it is 36.5 degrees or less, that means my thyroid gland is underactive, and I take 25 milligrams of T3. At mid-day, my temperature should be about 36.8-37.0 degrees Celsius. If it is lower, I take a second 25-milligram dose of T3 to keep the temperature around 37 degrees until 10 pm, when I go to bed. Of course, I also take supplements, as I explained before. I don't take only T4, because a lot of T4/T3 conversion problems that occur at my age keep me "hypothyroid" all day.

If my temperature is lower than 36.5 degrees in the morning, I assume that I didn't sleep well for various reasons, so I try to relax and take T3. I take my temperature again at mid-day to determine whether there are enough T3 molecules in my cells. My temperature should now be between 37.0 and 36.8 degrees. If I eat in a restaurant, my temperature usually drops because of the canola oil they use for cooking. In that case, if my plans include lunch in a restaurant, I take one or two dose of 400 IU of vitamin E (which is fat soluble) before lunch to help T3 enter my body cells. If my temperature has not dropped, my energy returns. I need coffee occasionally because my body temperature depends on what I eat during the day. The next morning, I can determine how much T3 I need—usually 50 micrograms during the day is enough.

Chapter 4

The Mystery Disease Is Called Hypothyroidism

In my opinion, hypothyroidism is a common phenomenon in the general population for two reasons: (1) the existing methods of diagnosis are based on the results of a thyroid-stimulating hormone (TSH) test only; and (2) the method of interpreting the test and waiting for the red asterisk is incorrect , which results in doctors missing the diagnosis of this disease. Because the diagnosis is missed, many diseases related to the phenomenon now called hypothyroidism begin to appear.

In my opinion, there are three forms of thyroid gland underactivity:

1. In young people with poor thyroid function, the pituitary gland secretes a high level of TSH, which allows for an easy diagnosis (Figure 4-1).

Name	Results	Units	Reference Range	Average Range
ESTRADIOL	less 70	pmol/L		
TSH	6.22	mIU/L	0.55-6.22	..........*
FT3	3.5	pmol/L	3.5-6.5	.*..........
FT4	17..5	pmol/L	10-20	........*...

Figure 4-1. A patient with a high TSH, a low FT3 (because of deficient 5'D enzyme conversion activity) and a high FT4 (because of a T4 overdose. This patient probably is producing many rT3 molecules. Compare with Figures 3-1. and 3-2. Abbreviations: TSH, thyroid-stimulating hormone; FT3, free triiodothyronine, 5'D, 5- 5'deiodinase; FT 4 free thyroxine;

2. In adults, latent hypothyroidism is identified by the position of the asterisk on your blood test results. Specifically, it appears in the low part of the average/normal range for T4 and T3 while your TSH levels are in the average/low range (Figure 4-2). This occurs when the hypothalamus has not sent instructions to the pituitary gland to secrete TSH to simulate thyroid activity. This is common in people who are very sick, in the presence of viral disease, or as a result of a drug treatment for brain disorders. Therefore, it can be quite challenging to make a diagnosis of thyroid hypoactivity using the TSH test alone.

Name	Results	Units	Reference Range	Average Range
FT4	0.95	ng/L	070-1.80	..*.........
FT3	94.47	ng/L	80-200	...*........
TSH	0.82	Miu/L	040-4.70	..*......

Figure 4-2. All thyroid values are apparently within the normal average range, but the very low TSH and T4 affect thyroid gland function, and the conversion to the active T3 hormone does not produce enough heat and energy to allow the body to function normally.

3. The T4/T3 conversion rate is disturbed because of a malfunction in enzyme 5'D activity. This is referred to as "low T3 syndrome." This situation appears when there is some type of inflammation in the body that affects 5'D function or a serious disease. As a result, your body temperature drops and TSH secretion increases to "coax" the gland into producing more T4 because the T3 blood level is not in the upper limit of the normal average range, as it should be (Figure 4-3).

3.5 ▼ **4**	6.5	4.0 pmol/L	T3- FREE
0.4 ▼ **3.02**	4.2	3.02 mIU/L	TSH
10 ▼ **14.7**	20	14.7 pmol/L	T4- FREE

Figure 4-3. The TSH is higher than 2 and the FT4 level is within normal limits, but the FT3 is very low due to defective 5'D enzyme function. These findings indicate low T3 syndrome.

The conversion of T4 to T3 is carried out by 5'D enzymes. There are different types of 5'D enzymes, and the activity of each is related to its day/night cycle; that is, some are active at night and others are active during the day. This enzyme is designed to remove one atom of iodine from a specific location in the T4 molecule to turn it into the active hormone, T3 (Figures 4-1 and 4-3). You may recall that T3 is essential to be alert and to feel and look good. When 5'D works well, a standard rate of conversion from T4 to T3 will occur and T3 will be secreted into the bloodstream. Under such circumstances, the asterisk indicating T3 activity might be in the upper third of the normal range. If 5'D activity is compromised (as I described previously), two situations may develop:

a. The production of a hormone called *rT3 (reverse T3),* an inactive hormone that disrupts the entry of T3 into the cell by attaching itself to T3 receptors on the membrane of the cell, mitochondrion, and nucleus, thereby blocking T3 activity. This results in the body temperature dropping below 36.8 degrees (98.2 degrees Fahrenheit) (Figures 3-2 and 4-1).

b. The entire enzymatic system stops because of a reduction in the production of ATP. A high level of rT3 has been found in many diseases. The test for rT3 is not carried out in health maintenance organization (HMO) clinics. In my opinion, however, it is not necessary.

Because T3 is responsible for a person's vitality, failure to properly diagnose hypothyroidism allows a syndrome to develop that includes a broad spectrum of complaints that vary from patient to patient, with each complaint varying in intensity. In this chapter, I want to put things in order and give the reader a complete understanding of the familiar yet mysterious disease called *hypothyroidism* and teach you how to interpret normal laboratory tests correctly. I will do this by comparing lab test results for individuals 40 years and older with values that are seen in adults aged 20 to 30 years (See Table 4-1). In the following pages, you will learn how to decode the lab results correctly. In children, the T3 value should be at the upper limit of normal, because the thyroid gland responds very well to TSH at that age. The T4/T3 conversion rate is also good, and 5'D activity is normal. The numbers are not important, because they vary among laboratories according to the method used to measure these variables. Of course, the situation is different for a child born with low T3 blood levels—for example, a child born to a woman with hypothyroidism. T3 needs to be at an optimal level to ensure the normal development of the body from birth to puberty.

If the asterisk is not high along the spectrum of possible values for a child, the child's brain will not function well, because T3 is needed for the brain to use glucose well. Otherwise, the child may develop a cognitive disorder such as attention-deficit/hyperactivity disorder (ADHD) or depression or abnormal behaviors during adolescence, as you will learn in Chapters 6 and 11. Between the ages of 20 and 30 years, T3 test results should also be at the upper limit of normal to provide enough T3 molecules for your body cells to function normally. **But disturbances in thyroid gland activity can appear at any age—from newborn to the third age.** An optimal level of T3 is necessary for the normal development of the human body during pregnancy, especially to activate embryonic stem cells and for their development into different types of body cells, for human reproduction to occur, and for the normal functioning of the brain and other organs. *Low T3 syndrome* is more common in women than men, because women tend to be under a greater amount of stress and are more frequently exposed to environmental stressors. With the information presented in medical literature today and the experience I have gained over the years, I understand that there is an "epidemic of chronic fatigue," which, according to the World Health Organization (WHO), is due to the fact that most people today are experiencing a "personal crisis in energy production"—in other words, a chronic deficiency of T3. A study from Stanford University in California, USA, reveals that out body temperatures have been on a continuous decline in the United States since the Industrial Revolution. To overcome fatigue, people often drink caffeine or other stimulant-containing substances. Caffeine causes many side effects, including heartburn. If this develops, the doctor may prescribe a drug to lower the acidity in the stomach. As a result, the stomach juices will not be able to extract vitamins and minerals from meats and other foods. Consequently, these nutrients (including vitamin

B12, folic acid, vitamin B6, and iron) will not be available to be absorbed from the intestines. Some time later, a lack of these essential nutrients may disrupt mitochondrial activity, reduce the T4/T3 conversion rate, and result in the appearance of disease.

A correct interpretation of laboratory tests: the lie in statistics

There appears to be a consistent inconsistency between patient complaints and the results of their laboratory tests. I have, for example, often heard this phrase from my patients: "Doctor, I don't feel well, but I was told that all my laboratory test results today are normal." What is the reason for this situation? First, it is crucial to understand how the average normal range is calculated for each laboratory test. Let's say a laboratory testing company finds a new method to measure the testosterone or some other biological substance. For example, the company uses its new laboratory testing method to measure testosterone levels because it is more effective or less expensive. To have its method accepted by other institutions, the company constructed an average normal range doing its test method in many individuals aged 20 to 70 years in the general population in specific regions of the globe. A statistical analysis of the lab values is carried out, and the results are plotted on a graph. The values result in a plot that appears in the shape of a bell (Figure 4-4). In my example, about 68.3% of the results fall in the high middle area of this "bell curve." That leaves a large group of people with high (to the right of the middle) and low (to the left of the middle) results. To include 95% of the tested population in this analysis, the statistician usually creates a *standard deviation*. In this case, the standard deviation is from two units above the maximum mean value (the peak of the bell curve) to two units below the maximum mean value. That means there are people with lower or higher testosterone results than those whose results are considered to be in the "average" range. Regarding testosterone, the high value is for young people and the low value for older people. Only when the lab result is lower or higher than average range will you see a red asterisk or other alarm sign, which indicates that the result is abnormal compared with the general population of 20- to 70-year-olds.

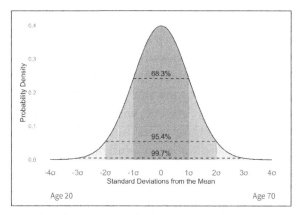

Figure 4-4. Statistical calculation of biological materials in a research laboratory.

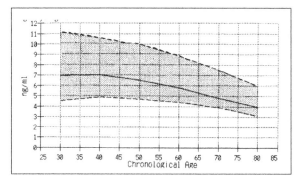

Figure 4-5. Testosterone levels start to decline gradually by the age of 30 and more rapidly at age 75.

This use of the red asterisk or other sign started in the laboratories of pharmaceutical companies during their investigations of new drugs. When this company discovers a new substance that is being considered as a treatment for human or animal diseases, it studies the physical proprieties of the substance first in an isolated cellular medium and later in animals. [Naturally, animals suffer from diseases similar to those in humans.] This process is essential before the substance is utilized in humans. For example, there are animals that suffer from high blood cholesterol or high glucose levels. First, the researcher performs a blood test on all the animals and then performs a statistical calculation of the cholesterol or sugar level in a group of laboratory animals of different ages. In the statistical processing, the results take on the shape of a bell, with low values for young animals and high values for mature animals. The researcher gives these animals the substance he is studying and expects to see a decrease in the level of cholesterol or sugar. Until a red asterisk appears or another sign on the low side, the researcher does not know if his research was successful and if the substance lowers the cholesterol (or sugar) level in the blood. When this method is transferred to humans, we can complain that something is wrong even before an alarm sign appears. Thus, lab blood tests provide two values: one high and the other low. If the asterisk is between these values, the doctor will think that you are fine despite your justified complaints. On some lab test reports, the letter H (for "high") or L (for "low") appears beside the value or a red asterisk may appear only to alert the doctor. Only when an alarm sign appears next to the value being monitored (cholesterol or glucose, for example) does the investigator or the doctor know something is wrong. That's how doctors have been taught to interpret laboratory results! Because the level of all biological substances changes from the optimal levels seen in individuals aged 20 to 30 years to a lower or higher level in older age groups,

I compare the blood test results for each patient with those seen between the ages of 20 and 30 years.

Another example should be mentioned regarding T3 or testosterone lab values: In a young population, these values are at the upper limit of normal; in older populations, they are at the lower limit of normal. What about the 30-year-old with a complaint of fatigue or decreased libido whose T3 or testosterone level is in the middle of the normal range? What happens if his values correspond with those seen at the age of 50? I'm sure he won't feel well, but because his test results are within normal limits, the doctor could miss the diagnosis if a red asterisk or an "L" does not appear. Therefore, it is a significant mistake to use this statistical method in humans. This is the main reason for the lack of diagnosis of many diseases and the proliferation of diseases.

The writer Mark Twain wrote about such phenomena: "There are three forms of lies: the lie itself, damned lies, and statistics." That's why I use a more accurate method to interpret hormonal tests (as well as other tests): I compare the current result with those that are seen at the age of 20 to 30 years (Table 4-1). Then I will see minimum changes of all biological substances. I want all biological materials to remain as they were at the age of 20 to 30 years so that the body functions well and you have no complaints. Not an easy task!

Therefore, *the interpretation of blood tests that is discussed in this book is according to the position of the asterisk on the scale of normal average values and in comparison with its position at the age of 20 to 30 years.* If the asterisk on a hormonal test (or test of any other biological substance) is not at the level seen in a 20- to 30-year-old, the patient may complain that something is wrong in his or her body. Their complaints will disappear only when the asterisk returns to the place it should be (at the age of 20 to 30 years). This can be achieved by taking a supplement containing substances that match the body's own biological substances—specifically hormones, vitamins, or minerals.

Another question is why do doctors rely solely on the results of a TSH test to determine if there is a disease in the thyroid gland. When I studied Harrison's *Principles of Internal Medicine* (which is read by every doctor who studies internal medicine), I learned the following about thyroid hormone tests: "In practice, the laboratory tests (fourth generation) of TSH are particularly sensitive, which can detect TSH levels as low as 0.004 μIU/L; but for practical purposes, tests sensitive to 0.1 μIU/mL are sufficient to determine whether TSH is suppressed, normal, or high"—that is, a TSH test is enough whether the patient has hyperthyroidism, normal thyroid activity, or hypothyroidism. That is the reason why HMOs (health maintenance organizations) used only TSH for the diagnosis of hypothyroidism. What if the patient's complaints appear before the alarm sign is seen next to TSH? That's why doctors use TSH test results without the results of FT4 and FT3. In fact, a TSH test only shows what is happening in the hypothalamus or pituitary gland and nothing more. The FT4 level tells if the thyroid gland is secreting enough T4 hormone, and the FT3 level shows if the 5'D enzyme is converting T4 to active T3 (as we will learn later). In fact, most of the medical research on the thyroid gland is carried out during treatment with only T4, and sometimes the conclusions are not clear because problems with the conversion of T4 into T3 or with the ability of T3 to enter the cells is not taken into account. I believe that doctors should be taught to assess the function of the thyroid gland correctly by measuring all of the hormones involved. This will allow for the examination, correct treatment, and prevention of many diseases (as we will see later).

TABLE 4-1. HORMONAL BLOOD LEVELS

Normal asterisk position at age 20-30	Asterisk position at age 40-50 complains	Asterisk position at age 60-70 complains
Normal Average Values	Lab Test	Lab Test
IGF-1 (3.8-26.5 pmol/L)	Obesity, high cholesterol, glucose, complaints	Obesity, high cholesterol, diabetes ,complaints
(..........*..)	(.............*..............)	(....*.................)
Cortisol (138-690 nmo;/L)	Mild stress	Severe stress obesity, other diseases
(....*................)	(.........*.........)	(.................*....)
&DHEA women (2.7-15.2 mmol/L)	Pre menopause, infertility, other disease	Menopause, infertility, other disease
(.................*....)	(.......*.............)	(....*..................)
DHEA men (2.7-15.2 mmol/L)&	Pre- andropause, complaints, other disease	Andropause, obesity, other diseases
(.................*....)	(.........*.............)	(....*..................)
TSH (0.4-4.2 mIU/ml)	Hypothyroidism	Hypothyroidism, other diseases
(...*..................)	(........*..........)	(......................*...)
Free-FT4 (10-20 pmol/L)	Hypothyroidism	Hyperthyroidism
(.........*..........)	(......*.............)	(....................)*
Free-FT4 (10-20 pmol/L)	Over dosage	Hypothyroidism
(.........*..........)	(..........*........)	(...*..................)
Free T3 3.5-6.5 pmol/L)	Hypothyroidism	Hyperthyroidism
(........*.......)	(.........*........)	(.....................)*
Free T3 3.5-6.5 pmol/L)	Low T3 Syndrome	Low T3 Syndrome
(........*.......)	(....*..............)	(....*.................)
PTH (Para-thyroid hormone)	Osteopenia, complaints, kidney disease	Osteoporosis, complains, kidney disease
(....*....................) 15-65 gram/ml	(........*...........)	(...............*......)

Vitamin D25 (50-100 ng/ml)&	Complaints, low immune system function	Over dose
(…….....*..........)	(….....*..................)	(…......................)*
LH women 50 year-old (5-25 IU/L)	peri-menopause, menstrual problems,	Menopause, complaints, other diseases
(…......*.............)	(…..*..........…........)	(…......…..............*....)
LH (5-25 IU/L) fertile women	Irregular periods, infertility, high exercise	Irregular periods, Polycystic Ovarian Syndrome
(….......*............) Days 18-24	(…*…................)	(….......................*....)
LH men (1.8-8.6 IU/L)	Complaints	Andropause, complaints
(….*..................)	(….........*..….......)	(….......….............*....)
FSH (< 5 mIU/ml)fertile women	complains,	Menopause, diminished ovarian reserve
(….*.................) Days 18-24	(…........*..…........)	(.....................*.....)
FSH fertile men (< 5 mIU/ml)	complains,	Andropause, testicles damage, disease
(…*.................)	(…........*..…........)	(.....................*.....)
Testosterone Total Men	Complains	Obesity, high cholesterol, complains
(.................*.....) (8.4-28.7 pm/L)	(…........*..............)	(…*.........................)
Bioavailable Testosterone	Reduce libido	Obesity, high cholesterol, complains
(.................*.....) 1.1-4.0 ng/ml	(…........*..............)	(…*.........................)
Testosterone women	Reduce libido	Hirsutism
(...........*............) (0.3-1.3 pm/L	(…*…...................)	(...........................)*
SHB Globulin (17-138 (nmol/L) man	Poor diet, complains, IBD, Renal disease	Complaints, autoimmune disease, cancer
(…......*............)	(….*.......…........)	(… ....*..)
Insulin (2-37.5 mIU/ml)	Diabetes type 2, belly obesity, over eat	Diabetes type 1, medications
(…*...................).	(..............*.........)	(*........................)

Estradiol women 50-400 pmol/L (.......*........)		Complaints, Menopause
over 50 year old		(...*......................)
Estradiol fertile women (50-400 pmol/L) (.......*........) days 18-24	Estradiol dominance, infertility, heavy cycle (..................)*	
Progesterone (5-20 ng/mlL &) (..........*.........) days 18-24 of cycle	Complaints, infertility, heavy periods (...*..............)	
Progesterone (5-20 ng/mlL) (..........*.........) 50 year old	Complaints. Perimenopause (......*..............)	Menopause (...*..................)
P/E2 Ratio X/0.x Days 18-24	Estradiol dominance, infertility, heavy cycle	Complains, Estradiol Dominance
More of 50	Less of 50	Less of 50
Estradiol men (70-180 pmol/L)	Prostate and Brest enlargement	Prostate enlargement cancer?
(....*..................)	(.......*.........)	(..........*.......)
Women 0.5-2.4 mmol/L Testosterone	hirsutism	low libido
(........*.......)	(..........*.......)	(..*.............)
Prolactin men (20-400micro gram/L	Stress Low libido	Hypothyroidism
(..*..................)	(......*........)	(...........*....)
Prolactin women less of 25 ngmm/L	Decrease libido, stress	Hypothyroidismn Infertility
(..*..................)	(......*........)	(..............*...)

Hormonal Changes from age 20-70 and diseases development.
Final diagnosis may be done according with the medical recommendations.
Warning: taken DHEA or Testosterone may raise the level of Estradiol;
Take Anti-aromatase supplement like indol-3*carbinol and others.
Check Estradiol every 3 months

TABLE 4-2. GENERAL BLOOD

AGE 20-30	AGE 40-50	AGE 60-70
Normal Average Values	Lab Test	Lab Test
Glucose (70-100 mg/dl	Pre-diabetes	Diabetes
(...*...............)	(...............*.......)	(...................*....)
Hemoglobin A1C(3.5-5.7%)	Pre-diabetes	Diabetes
(...*...................)	(..............*.........)	(....................*...)
Kidney Function		
Urea(17-43 mg/dl)	Dehydration? Disease	Kidney Disease
(...*..............)	(.......*........)	(..............*...)
Creatinine(0.5-1.3 mg/dl	Kidney Disease?	Kidney Disease
(...*.............)	(.......*........)	(..............*...)
Uric acid (3.5-8.2 mg/dl)	Kidney Disease?	Disease
(...*.............)	(...........*.............)	(...................*....)
Liver Function	Disease	Liver Disease
(...*...lower value)	(.........*.........)	(...............*.)
LDH	complains, Fatty Liver	Liver Disease, Stroke, Heart MI' Hemolysis
(...*...lower value)	(.........*.........)	(...............*.)
(GOT(10-37 IU/L)	complains	Liver, bleeding, heart, infection
(..*................)	(.........*.........)	(...............*.)
ALT(GPT) (0-37 IU/L	complains	Heart, muscle, liver
(..*.............37)	(.........*.........)	(..............*..)
Alkaline Phosph (30-80 mg/dl)	Low-Protein Diet	Liver, alcohol, anemia, bone
(....*..........)	(....*.......-......)	(...............*.)
GGT(0-57 IU/L)	complains	Liver, kidney, bone
(.*..................)	(....*.............)	(.............*..)
Bilirubin Direct(0-0.3 mg/dl	complains	Liver, gall bladder
(..*...........)	(.......*.........)	(...............*.....)

Bilirubin Total (1.9-0.3	complains	Bleeding, anemia
(...........*..........)	(...........*........)	
GENERAL PROTEINS		
Albumin 3.5-5.2 g/dl	Low-Protein Diet	Liver, Kidney Disease
(.........*.....)	(.....*..........)	(..*...............)
Total Protein 6.6-8.3 g/dl	Low-Protein Diet	Liver Kidney Disease
(.........*.........)	(..........*.......)	(..*................)
Globulin 2.1-3.4 g/dl	Immune Disease	Liver, Kidney Disease
(.........*.........)	(...........*.....)	(..*................)
Globulin 2.1-3.4 g/dl	Bowel Disease	Cancer Multiple Myeloma
(..............*...)	(....*...........)	(................*..)
Different fats types		
Cholesterol, total 120-200 mg/dl	Disease? Over eating Carbs	Disease? Overeating Carbs
(...*..............)	(..........*.......)	(...............*..)
Triglycerides, less than150 mg/dl	over eating carbs	Overeating carbs
(...*.............)	(..........*.......)	(...............)*
LDL Cholesterol < 130 mg/dl	Disease?	Disease? Overeating Carbs
130(...*.............)	(..........*.......)	(...............)*
HDL Cholesterol more than 40mg/dl	Disease?	Disease
(.............*...)	(........*.......)	(...............)*
PSA,(0-4ng/ml	Prostate Enlargement	Cancer?
(....*................)	(..........*.......)	(...............)*
Anti-TPO/ Ag Must be(0)	Hashimoto disease	Hashimoto disease
(*....................)	(............*....)	(.............*..)
Anti TSH Receptor Ag	Graves' Disease	Graves' Disease
(*....................)must be 0	9.........*.......)	(............*)

Final diagnosis must be done with other studies according with the medical recommendations

TABLE 4-3. VITAMIN AND MINERALES

AGE 20-30	AGE 40-50	AGE 60-70	COMMENTS
Iron(35+175 microG/dl	disease Anemia?	Anemia	high dosage. Disease
(.........*.........)	(......*...........)	(...*..........)	(........... *.)
B12(187-500 pg/dl)	disease?	Anemia	high dosage
(.......*..........)	(......*...........)	(...*..........)	(.............)*
Folic Acid(3.10-20.5 ng/dl)	disease	disease	high dosage
(.........*..........)	(......*...........)	(...*..........)	(.............)*
Ferritin(21.8-175(ng/dl	disease Anemia?	Disease Anemia	high dosage
(.......*........)	(......*...........)	(...*..........)	(.............)*
Sodium(134-146)meg/L	Disease, diuretics	Disease, drink much water	high intake, low fluids
(........*............)	(...*..........)	(...*..........)	(.............)*
Potassium (3.5-5.30(meq/L	Diuretics	Diuretics	Blood Hemolysis
(........*...........)	(......*...........)	(...*..........)	(.............)*
Calcium(8.8-10.6mg/dl	disease	disease	disease Hypercalcemia
(........*...........)	(......*...........)	(*...... ......)	(.............)*
Phosphorus(2.5-4.5 mg/dl	disease	disease	disease
(........*...........)	(......*...........)	(..*..........)	(.............)*

Final diagnosis must be done with other studies according to the medical recommendations

TABLE 4-4. BLOOD CELLS COUNTS

AGE 20-30	AGE 40-50	AGE 60-70	COMMENTS
WBC	Weak immune system	Infection' blood cancer	Measure the nro of WBC
(..........*............).	(...*.................)	(...................)*	כדוריות לבנות =WBC
RBC	Anemia	Disease	Count nro of RBC
(..........*............).	(...*.................)	(...................)*	כדוריות אדומות=RBC
HGB	Anemia	Disease	counts the HGB red levels
(..........*............).	(...*.................)	(...................)*	
HCT	anemia	Disease	Measure the HGB in blood
(..........*............).	(...*.................)	(...................)*	
MCV	iron deficiency	B12 anemia	Mean red cells volume
(..........*............).	(...*.................)	(...................)*	
MCH	iron deficiency	B12 anemia	HGB concentration in RBC
(..........*............).	(...*.................)	(...*.............)	
MCHC	iron deficiency	B12 deficiency	measures HGB in RBC
(..........*............).	(...*.................)	(...................)*	
PLT(טסיות)	Disease-Drugs (bleeding)	Clots formation (pills)	for blood coagulation
(..........*............).	(...*.................)	(...................)*	
RDW-	Anemia by iron loss	B12 deficiency	the mean RBC volume
(..........*............).	(...*.................)	(...................)*	

PDW	? Problems with blood coagulation	disease,	PLT Volume distribution
(.........*.............).	(...*.................)	(....................)*	
PCT	person with infection	Severe Infection	Procalcitonin (PCT)
(...*....................).	(..........*..........)	(....................)*	
MPV	? Problems with blood coagulation	disease,	Mean PLT volume
(...........*............).	(...*.................)	(....................)*	
Nucleated RBC	cell cancer? after severe bleeding	disease, cancer	Nucleus in the RBC
0	(...........*.........)	(....................)*	
White Cells Differential			
Neutrophils	Weak immune system	Infection	Types of WBC
(..........*............).	(...*.................)	(....................)*	
Lymphocytes % 30.0 %	Weak immune system	viral Infection	Types of WBC
(..........*............).	(...*.................)	(....................)*	
Monocytes % 6.1 %	Weak immune system	viral Infection	Type of WBC
(..........*............).	(...*.................)	(....................)*	
Eosinophils	Food allergy	severe food allergy	Type of WBC
(...*....................).	(..........*..........)	(....................)*	
Basophils	Suspect Food allergy, parasites....	parasites, fungi and cancer	Type of WBC
(...*....................).	(..........*..........)	(....................)*	
Coagulation			

PT(11-13.5 second	Drugs, bleeding, liver	clots more quickly than normal	Time to appear a clot
(…….*.........)	(…..................*…..)	(…*.................)	
INR 0.8-11 sec.	Risk for dangerous blood clots	drugs, liver disease	Time blood to clot
1.1 second	less 1 sec	4-5 sec.	
PTT(25-35 sec)	Bleeding, liver disease	Risk of coagulation	Time blood to clot
(……..*.........)	(…..................*…..)	(..*….................)	

Final diagnosis must be done with other studies according with the medical recommendations

Each biological substance has its own range of normal values at age 20 to 30 years (see Table 4-1 to 4-4). If a black asterisk appears among them, the doctor will declare that you are healthy, having compared your results with those of the entire population. My approach is different, however, because I compare your current lab results with those of individuals 20 to 30 years of age. At age 20, the TSH p.e. the asterisk should be in the lower limit of average values (that is, less than 2.0). If TSH is marked by a black asterisk and its value is going up but is still below the higher values, that means the thyroid gland is "sick," and TSH is pushing it to produce more T4 and T3. I don't need to wait until the red asterisk appears. This is why you may not feel well and still hear your doctor tell you that your test results are normal.

Another consideration should be noted regarding T3: Its value should be in the upper limit of the normal range in a young population and in the lower limit of normal in an older population. What is happening in a person who, at the age of 30, has a "low normal" T3 level corresponding to that of an individual who is 50 years old? I'm sure he won't feel well. Because the test results are within the limits of average values, however, the doctor will treat the patient as though his reading was within normal limits. This small movement of the T3 asterisk down means that the enzyme 5'D is not doing its job. Therefore, it is a significant mistake to use this method of measurement in humans. This is the main reason for the failure to diagnose many diseases and for the proliferation of disease. The patient complaints will resolve only when the TSH and the T3 returned to the 20-30 column .

You will be alert to any change in the different blood studies when they began to be part of the column 20-30, that means that you need to make some change in your lifestyle. Whether you complain or not, a disease may develop and you must prevent this by consulting with your doctor to return an abnormal value to age 20-30 column.

When the proper level of thyroid hormones is achieved, the enzymes will function properly at any age because they will be getting energy, or a vitamin or mineral return to the column 20-30 you will feel better because the mitochondria is producing energy as indicated by the rate of blood flow in the body, the activity of the digestive system and the sexual and reproductive systems, the ability to think and concentrate, mood and motivation, muscular conditioning, and what not. Otherwise, enzymatic activity in other glands will not be as strong as it could be, and they will secrete fewer hormones due to a lack of energy. Thus, an inadequate T3 output, a low vitamin or minerals level is frequently accompanied by hormonal disorders in other glands.

When a specific area of the body does not receive enough T3, the body temperature drops and symptoms of poor hormonal activity appear. These symptoms will vary from person to person and extend from the hair roots on the head to the toenails. I propose calling this common 21st century phenomenon a "personal energy crisis," because the lack of T3 worldwide seems to be permanent. The loss of energy due to the lack of T3 has led to the widespread use of coffee and other stimulants, as well as to the increased use of industrial fats and drugs.

A global fatigue epidemic after the COVID-19 pandemic has being attributed for many researchers to environmental factors and various diseases. As I have explained so far, however, the reasons for the gradual decrease in body temperature are within us: a "personal crisis in energy production" due to damage to the mitochondrial enzyme 5' deiodinase (5'D for short) affecting their ability to function and the causing a decrease in the natural production of T3. When we return natural substances—minerals, vitamins, natural saturated fats, and natural hormones—to the levels the mitochondria require to function optimally, the amount of T3 and heat in the body will return to their normal course. Think carefully. You may disagree with me, but if you make a personal attempt to reduce the amount of these toxic substances in your diet for 2 weeks, you will see a change for the better, as I did. Of course, I don't want to bring more problems into your life than you already have. It all depends on the level of health you desire. I chose to live a healthy life until I reach 120 years. I prefer to act, to enjoy my life and not disturb the body's natural functions.

As you can tell from what you have read so far, production of the primary thyroid hormone—the T3 hormone—can go wrong in any of the "stations" described in Figure 3-1: the hypothalamus, the pituitary gland, the thyroid gland itself, in blood proteins, and in the cell membranes (if their T4 or T3 receptors are blocked by rT3 or other material). The most frequent issue causing the most problems is the 5'D enzyme. Many diseases, as well as medications and other substances, can interfere with 5'D activity in the liver and kidneys, thereby lowering T3 levels in the blood. Many of the factors that affect 5'D activity (and increase the production of rT3) are known and are documented in the medical literature. They include the following:

1. Some inflammatory processes, mainly in patients with diabetes.
2. Deficiency in iron, vitamin D, selenium, iodine, magnesium, zinc, and copper.
3. Old age and serious diseases, including cancer (mainly because of the effect of therapeutic drugs).
4. Low testosterone levels in men; low estradiol and progesterone levels in women and men.
5. Many drugs used to treat heart rhythm disorders, high blood pressure, and high cholesterol; also, birth control drugs, steroids (for example, prednisone), and many others.
6. Liver diseases, including fatty liver, and metabolic syndrome
7. Viruses: for example, COVID-19, HIV, Epstein-Barr virus (EBV), cytomegalovirus (CMV). and hepatitis virus.
8. Kidney or liver disease of any type.
9. Obesity is caused by eating too many carbohydrates before going to bed or during the day.
10. Stress. This is an image that controls our lives. You see it on TV or read about it in the newspapers. Chronic stress increases blood levels of the hormone cortisol, which paralyzes 5'D activity. As a result, the conversion of T4 to T3 is impaired, rT3 levels rise, the T3 level in the blood falls to the lower part of the standard curve, and many enzymatic systems become disturbed. The major damage is to the 5'D enzyme, the mitochondria (which produce fewer energy particles), and thyroid function. The cells use less sugar or cholesterol to produce energy and heat. Thus, a woman with an underactive thyroid gland due to stress or a difficult birth will have a lower T3 level, which may put her at risk for depression or make it difficult for her to recover from depression. It will also make it difficult for any individual to control diabetes or cholesterol levels or recover from kidney failure, heart failure, and other serious diseases. In men, prolonged stress

may also cause depression or the development of a disease.

11. If you have already been diagnosed with hypothyroidism, your doctor may have made the diagnosis on the basis of a high TSH reading. You will receive the medically accepted treatment of T4 only (UthyroxTM, Eltroxin®, and Synthroid®) at a dose of 50 micrograms per day. After a certain period of time, however, you will go to the doctor again because you will still have symptoms. However, the doctor will show you that your thyroid hormones are balanced because the TSH level is within normal limits. Any of several scenarios may then occur:

a. You get frustrated by your symptoms continuing even though your hormones are allegedly "balanced." Your doctor increases your T4 dose to 100 micrograms per day. This disturbs the 5'D enzyme function, however, and results in a higher rT3 level.

b. You think the pill that contains the T4 hormone is causing your "side effects," so you replace it with another medication that contains only T4 or you look for a "better" medicine. I've heard all of these potential "solutions" from patients.

c. What is actually happening is that the 5'D enzyme is not producing enough T3 because the 5'D lacks one or more of the substances I described before or because it is producing too much rT3, which blocks the entry of T3 into the cells. How will you discover the cause? The T3 level in your blood is not in the upper third of the normal range, the T4/T3 conversion rate is low, and your body temperature is lower than 36.8 to 37.0 degrees Celsius (98.6-98.2 degrees Fahrenheit) most of the day. The 5'D enzyme has declared a "slow-down strike." As a result, it produces considerably more rT3 than T3, thereby disrupting T3 activity in different areas of the cell: its outer membrane, its nuclear membrane, or its mitochondrial membrane. This is what happens when the patient receives more of 50 micrograms of T4 before anyone finds out whether the 5'D is working properly (see case reports in Chapter 6).

Why don't doctors diagnose hypothyroidism at the required frequency?

For tree important reasons:

1. Doctors use the TSH test only according with Dr Harrison's recommendation and wait for a red asterisk or other sign to appear near or above the high limit to make a diagnosis of hypothyroidism or at the lower limit to make a diagnosis of hyperthyroidism and normal when the results are between them.
2. 2.The usual lab decoding that compares the results with those of the wide range of 20- to 70-year-old age population.
3. .3 The active hormone T3 is not measured. This, as I explained, is essential. Any change from a higher level to a lower one affects the production of heat and energy in the cell and increases the risk of developing diseases (Figure 4-6).

Name of Test	Results	Units	Average Range	Asterisk Placement
Trijodothyronine Free FT3	3.72	pmol/L	3.50-6.50	..(*...........)..

Figure 4-6. The T3 level in a 25-year-old woman with many symptoms of hypothyroidism and a severe menstrual disorder. Her body temperature is 36.2 degrees Celsius (97.2 degrees Fahrenheit). I requested a T3 study; the result was considered normal. Because the FT3 level was in the lower average range, however, a deficit in the conversion of T4 to T3 resulting from a malfunction in 5'D activity was suspected.

The normal values for thyroid hormones appear in Figure 4-7.

Name	Results	Normal Range
TSH	lower than 2 mIU/L	0.4(.. *...........)4.2
Free T4	15 pmol/L	10(.....*.......)20
Free T3	5.8 pmol/L	3.5(.........*....)6.5

Figure 4-7. The correct diagnosis of a thyroid hormone disorder is made according to the position of the asterisk within the normal range. To feel good, the levels of these hormones should be different: T3 should be in the high range (which indicates a good T4/T3 conversion rate), and T4 should be in the middle range. The thyroid gland secretes this hormone regularly during the night. In this reading, the TSH is less than 2—a sign that the thyroid gland is responding well to TSH activity.

Hormone	Amount	Range	Asterisk Placement
Free T4	14.60 pmol/L	(9.00-19.00)	(.....*......)
Testosterone	19.06 pmol/L	(8.40-28.70)	(.....*......)
Free T3	5.5 pmol/L	(2.66-5.70)	(............*.)
TSH	1.95 pmol/L	(0.35-4.94)	(...*........)
CRP	<5.0	(0.00-5.70)	

Figure 4-8. The blood test results for a 34-year-old man with a temperature of 37 degrees Celsius (98.6 degrees Fahrenheit). T3 is in the upper third of the normal range, and T4 is in the middle range. The TSH is less than 2, which puts it in the lower third of the normal range. Testosterone should be in the upper third of the average readings. but it is lower here. The patient's complaint was related to this finding.

What could go wrong with the hormonal mechanism that produces heat and energy in the body? As I described earlier, various failures and blockages can occur at different stations during the long and complex process of producing T3. As we can see in the following illustration, several scenarios can take place:

1. The hypothalamus can get damaged. If so, the pituitary gland will not secrete TSH. This usually occurs as a result of

an inflammatory process in the body, aging, or the administration of a drug used to treat brain diseases (see Chapter 6). It can also occur when there is a severe viral or bacterial infection, for example, by COVID-19. As a result, TSH levels will decrease. Any hospitalized patient with a severe infection or a serious illness will have a body temperature lower than 36.5 degrees and a low "normal" level of TSH and thyroid hormones. Their doctors are usually so focused on treating the patient's primary disease, however, that they fail to address any thyroid-specific issues.

Test Name	Results	Units	References Values	Normal Range
ESTRADIOL	678.5	pmol/L	98.1-571	.....*.......
PROGESTERONE	53.36	nmol/L	5.82-75.90	..........*...
FT4	1.05	ng/dL	0.80-1.90	.........*..
FT3	2.6	ng/dL	2.0-4.40	..*..........
TSH	0.597	mIU/L	0.270-4.200	.*..........

Figure 4-9. Thyroid panel for R.T. About a year ago, R.T., 28-year-old woman, got sick from the COVID-19 virus. Shortly after her recovery, a new disease developed that made her so weak that she had great difficulty functioning at home. Her laboratory test results revealed the cause of this weakness: low thyroid hormones levels. This reflects the fact that the conversion of T4 to T3 is also affected by low TSH levels. The decline in TSH may reflect diminished activity in the hypothalamus or the pituitary gland in response to toxins secreted by the virus or a change in cytokine activity (cytokines are proteins secreted by white blood cells called lymphocytes, which stimulate the immune system to produce antibodies against an invader, such as viruses). A similar situation can occur in patients who become infected with other viruses such as the Epstein-Barre virus, cytomegalovirus, or one of the hepatitis viruses. This patient did not recover after the active period of the virus had passed. Her body temperature ranged from 35.4 degrees to 36.2 degrees Celsius. In her case, other hormonal systems were not affected. Her menstrual cycle was normal, as indicated by her estradiol and progesterone levels and her P/2E ratio, which was greater than 50 (see below). The thyroid gland was not producing enough T4, however, proba-

bly because it had been attacked by the virus itself. This resulted in inflammation after exposure to free radicals, viral infections, or other conditions.

2 .The hypothalamus and the pituitary gland were either par-
alyzed by viral toxins or damaged by free radicals produced
by the virus. This could have prevented the pituitary gland
from receiving operating instructions from the hypothalamus. In either case, the hypothalamus is not producing
enough TSH and, consequently, her thyroid gland has not
responded (Figure 4-10). It is possible that the viral toxin
only affects hypothalamic activity associated with the thyroid gland and, perhaps, other areas of the brain associated
with taste or smell. These patients are at high risk for producing low levels of T4, T3, and TSH. Because the immune
system does not have enough energy (that is, enough T3 to
produce antibodies against the virus, the patient develops
pneumonia, for example. The patient is then treated with
antibiotics alone and will require more energy than usual to
cope with the increased immune system activity. To reduce
mortality among these patients, I recommend adding 25 to
50 micrograms of T3 to the antibiotic treatment to improve
the body's immune response against the virus.

3. In patients with Hashimoto's thyroiditis, the immune system attacks the thyroid gland and impairs its activity. This
disease involves an inflammatory process; as an autoimmune disease, it produces many lymphocyte cells in the
gland, thereby reducing its secretion of T4 and the rate of
conversion of T4 to T3. Thus, it is wise to give T3 instead of
T4 alone.

4. Disturbance in 5'D enzyme activity: As we explained earlier, 5'D enzyme activity can stop for many reasons: a lack of
certain vitamins and minerals, a low level of sex hormones,
or a high dose of T4 and a high rT3 level (Figure 4-11). In

geriatric cases and individuals with various diseases, drugs might delay the conversion of T4 to T3, causing the T3 level in the blood to decrease. Thus, this enzyme is at the central junction of all medical problems related to the diagnosis of hypothyroidism.

5. T4 and T3 are not absorbed in the intestines. Various diseases in the digestive system accompany this phenomenon. Laboratory tests show a low level of T4 and T3, even though the patient is being treated with these hormones. Maybe the patient didn't take the pills with water after an overnight fast or took them with food or coffee, which would prevent them from being absorbed. For this reason, I recommend advising patients who have a history of gastrointestinal disturbance to put the pill under the tongue so the medication can be absorbed through the oral mucosa.

Test Name	Results	Units	Reference Values	Normal Range
TSH	0.855	mIU/L	0.270-4.200	...*..........
Free T4	0.87	ng/dL	0.80-1.90	*............
Free T3	3.5	pg/dL	2.0-4.4	.........*...

Figure 4-10. These are the results for a woman taking T4 50 micrograms per day and T3 25 micrograms per day. Her FT4 level is very low, probably because of inadequate absorption of T4. She told me that she is taking both pills early in the morning with water. I recommended putting both pills under her tongue.

6. The mitochondria do not produce energy because various drugs have damaged them, for example, cholesterol-lowering drugs that reduce coenzyme Q10 (Figures 4-9, 4-10, 4-11, 4-12).

Test Name	Results	Units	Reference Values	Normal Range
TSH	0.83	mIU/L	0.4-4.7	...*........
Free T4	1.25	ng/dL	0.7-1.8	.........*...
Free T3	84.48	ng/dL	80-200	..*..............

Figure 4-11. A 57-year-old man taking statins complains about weakness and muscle pain. The FT4 asterisk is in the middle of the average range, which means that the thyroid gland is producing enough T4. The TSH is low, however, as is the T3 level. One posible explanation for this is that statins affect 5'D activity or the mitochondria are not producing enough energy because of low coenzyme Q10 levels. Note that the physician did not take the patient's body temperature (Figures 4-10 to 4-12). Some doctors do not recommend Q10 supplementation.

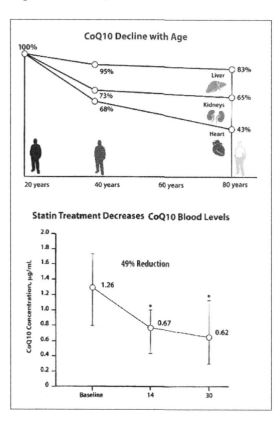

Figure 4-12. Statins reduce coenzyme Q10 levels in blood by 50%. It also decreases with age. From: Disease Prevention and Treatment (Life Extension).

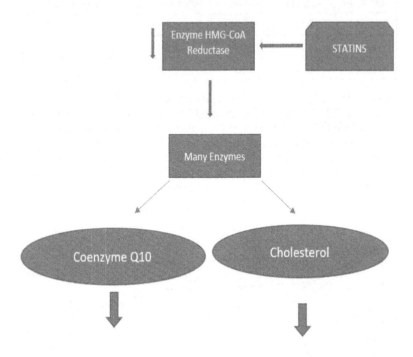

Figure 4-13. The enzymatic systems that produce cholesterol in the liver. Cholesterol-lowering drugs can paralyze an enzyme called HMG-CoA reductase. The final result: a decrease in the level of cholesterol in the blood, but also a decrease in the amount of coenzyme Q10, which is necessary for the mitochondria to create energy under the influence of T3 (see Figure 4-13).

Thymus: Role for T3 in improving immune activity

The thymus gland is where the cells of the immune system differentiate to carry out specific actions against viruses, bacteria, and cancer cells. This is where lymphocytes known as natural killer cells (NK cells) are produced. T3 ensures the flow of energy to the thymus gland so that it can function in the best way possible. It also activates immune cells to attack bacteria, viruses, and cancer cells. The activity of the immune system decreases with age, however, along with the level of essential hormones. For example, the thymus depends on T3, together with IGF-1 and the sex hormones, to produce its own hormones: thymosin, thymopoietin, and thymosin.

In conclusion: It seems to me that the expected low T3 syndrome is much more common than has been published in the literature. We see that the body's energy production is complex and combines many processes. There are many stops along the way, and various factors can disrupt this process. Hormone replacement therapy with thyroid hormones (T3) can prevent many diseases and revive the activity of the immune system, as well as reverse the lack of energy particles and decrease in temperature. Therefore, it is more important to think of the thyroid gland as a complete system rather than a single gland that only produces T4 and releases it into the bloodstream.

The conversion of T4 to T3 takes place in the cells regularly to keep the body temperature stable and in the mitochondria to create energy particles. The mitochondria appear to be the spring of a healthy life. Therefore, maintaining their regular activity for many years and keeping T3 levels in the upper third of the normal range can improve the quality of life at any age. Frequently it is necessary to balance other hormones in the body (see Chapter 2). Hormones activate appropriate segments of your DNA and refresh all cell components, including the 5'D enzymes. Therefore, we will need to maintain optimal levels of the main hormones throughout life. Every time you feel unwell, take your temperature, and you will see why! In Chapter 1, which discusses the mitochondria, you can find what the mitochondria need to function well. In this chapter, you'll find the optimal level of every hormone (Table 4-1).

Chapter 5

Your Complaints are Due to the Lack of T3 in Your Body Tissues

Because of the complex activity of the T3 hormone, any decrease in the T3 blood level can disrupt cell activity. Also, an optimal supply of ATP energy has a decisive effect on enzymatic activity, which is also essential to satisfy the cell's energy needs and must be available in every cell in every organ without interruption. This is why T3 is vital for the body to function normally and why it affects the body in a multi-system way. When T3 levels in the blood or in the cells are not optimal, multifaceted symptoms begin to appear. The list of patient complaints is long, and all of them indicate low levels of T3, together with the sex hormones. I gathered these data through my experience as a physician and cardiologist with a large number of patients. You will continue to function, your body temperature will continue to reach 36.5 degrees Celsius daily, and your symptoms will be tolerable. According to my experience, you will function excellently with a body temperature of 37 degrees. Your body temperature changes with environmental factors, diet, stress, high estradiol and cortisol levels, and other factors, as I mentioned earlier. You can temporarily overcome the situation, of course. However, I recommend that if you feel something is wrong, mark your symptoms (as described below) or look for the list of symptoms and the end of the book and take your temperature as described before:

• **Alertness and energy:** No matter when you wake up, if you feel tired when you get up and this feeling continues throughout the day, along with a decrease in the speed of your body movements and speech, it may mean that you are not producing enough energy. You may experience prolonged and unexplained fatigue, a lack of sleep or a desire for a lot of sleep, the need to rest at noon, weakness, prolonged fatigue after physical activity involving little effort, a decrease in selfishness, the inability to concentrate, snoring, and a reduced knee-jerk or Achilles tendon reflex.

• **Low metabolism:** You will complain about weight gain or the inability to lose weight despite diet and exercise, as well as an increase in body fat and symptoms of the metabolic syndrome, overweight or weight loss, and increased or decreased appetite.

• **Blood circulation:** T3 causes the small blood vessels to expand, thereby increasing blood flow to the internal organs and skin while reducing the diastolic blood pressure. This ensures an adequate supply of nutrients to the internal organs and the skin, as well as the rapid removal of the waste and water created in them. During a T3 deficiency, you will see edema in the face (particularly around the eyes) or in the legs and experience cold limbs, hypersensitivity to cold, cold sweats, night sweats, and profuse sweating during the day, high cholesterol, increased glucose levels, increased blood pressure, and heart disease.

• **Tendency toward infections:** When you experience a high frequency of flu and infections in the lungs and sinuses due to lack of immunoglobulin A; skin infections (such as psoriasis); infections caused by Helicobacter pylori bacteria in the in the stomach and cancer, or Candida bacteria, typically in the mouth, throat, gut, or vagina; fungal infection in the toenails (athlete's foot); or recurrent infections in the urine—this may be a sign that the immune system has weakened, possibly because a low T3 blood level.

• **Diseases in the digestive system:** Many patients complain of digestive disorders caused by food allergies. The intestines require a lot of energy to carry out their tasks; that's why you can develop constipation, anal fissures, hemorrhoids, diarrhea, lactose sensitivity, celiac disease, gluten sensitivity, irritable bowel syndrome (IBS), swallowing disorders, a feeling that food is stuck in the throat, and gas, as well as heartburn, a reflux disorder, a stomach ulcer, and pancreatitis. Many of these disorders are related to food sensitivity or drinking a lot of coffee. Check your temperature!

• **Vascular diseases:** What about fats? There is an excellent debate about whether saturated fats cause heart disease or unsaturated fats improve the lipid profile. Some "experts" recommend canola oil or other vegetable (polyunsaturated) oils(PUFAs). I know that I can eat animal fats if my hormonal system is balanced as you see in Chapter 2—in other words, if the T3 and other hormone levels are in the normal upper limit. When this occurs, the mitochondria use cholesterol and sugar to produce energy, and T3 rapidly reduces glucose and cholesterol levels in the blood. I only use olive oil. A decrease in the production of nitric oxide by the inner layer of arterial cells allows cholesterol to accumulate in the arterial walls (Figure 5-1 and 5-2).

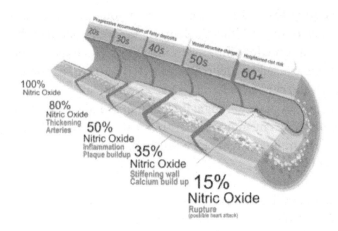

Figure 5-1. A decrease in nitric oxide levels in the endothelium promotes the development of arteriosclerosis. Available at: https://www.victorymenshealth. com/what-to-know-about-nitric-oxide/ This link may lead to you information that can help you increase your production of nitric oxide.

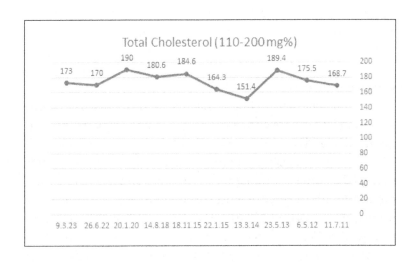

Figure 5-2. My cholesterol level over several years after treatment with natural hormones.

The layer of cholesterol plaque is probably related to the lack of energy being produced in the endothelial cells and the oxidation of cholesterol by free radicals, which may be reduced by T3 treatment. Patients exhibiting this phenomenon probably have suboptimal amounts of T3 (and other hormones) in the blood.

A decrease in the level of nitric oxide coincides with a decrease in many hormones after age 40 to 50 years and a rise in sugar and cholesterol levels. Therefore, the hormonal balance can lower cholesterol and sugar levels to below the upper line and renew the secretion of nitric oxide. Another factor to consider is a high homocysteine level as a cause of arterial blockage, which is not taken into account in general medicine (see case study in Chapter 6).

• **Food allergy:** Food allergies are related to interactions between the immune system and food allergens. Allergies may involve the release of histamine, which causes skin irritation, rashes, asthma, fatigue, diarrhea, weakness and other symptoms of allergy. This substance has been found in many foods. When a large amount of histamine is released, the cells that release it make contact with the cells of the immune system. An inflammatory reaction results in the blood vessels to dilate and typical symptoms of allergy to develop in the skin, digestive system, muscles and other body areas. Patients who develop these reactions tend to have high blood estradiol levels which, in turn, suppress the activity of a blood enzyme called diamine oxidase (DAO), which immediately neutralizes the histamine. High estradiol levels also raise the level of histamine in the blood, thereby creating a closed circuit of *histamine* ⟶ *estradiol* ⟶ *histamine*. A high level of estradiol also suppresses the conversion of T4 to T3. Thus, many digestive symptoms may be associated with hypothyroidism and/or high estradiol levels. When we treat patients exhibiting these two problems (excessive estradiol and hypothyroidism), I also treat first any allergies that I find. The hippocampus manages these allergic reactions. It saves in its memory cells information about every food that you eat and sends an alert if it is wrong for you.

The hippocampus is listening all the time! When we consume a food a second time, but its design or content has changed somewhat, the hypothalamus will warn us by triggering diarrhea, vomiting, a runny nose, a skin rash, asthma, or weakness.

• **Effect on the heart:** The heart requires a lot of energy to contract and relax properly. An inadequate amount of coenzyme Q10 in the mitochondria will prevent heart cells from producing enough energy to contract or relax. Q10 levels may become inadequate in patients who take statin drugs for a long time. Statins reduce the rate of T4/T3 conversion and lower T3 blood levels. This will cause the heart to expand and show an increase in atrial volume and frequency of ventricular and atrial arrhythmias. Blood output decreases due to heart failure, and several types of arrhythmias may occur. Shimabara and colleagues reported this finding of low T3 hormone levels in patients with heart failure and ventricular tachyarrhythmias (see case report in Chapter 6). Sometimes these types of arrhythmias appear after bypass surgery, valve replacement surgery, or another surgical procedure. The main reason for this condition is a decrease in energy production due to low T3 and Q10 levels (Figure 5-3).

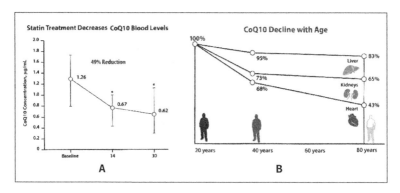

Figure 5-3. Comparison of change in Q10 enzymes with or without statin therapy. a: The Q10 level decreases by 50% after statin treatment. b: Natural change in Q10 level over lifetime. Taken from Disease Prevention and Treatment. Life Extension.

There may be several reasons for any cardiac event resulting from blocked arteries; for example, a decrease in T3 and sex hormone levels derived from cholesterol (Figure 5-4), causing an increase in cholesterol and glucose in the blood when several glands stop utilizing cholesterol to secrete their hormones.

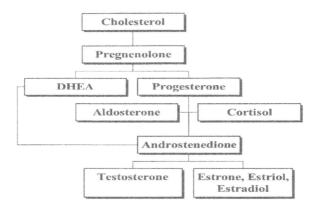

Figure 5-4. Hormones created from cholesterol.

Also, an increase in the amino acid homocysteine (due to drinking a lot of coffee) may result in a deficiency in vitamin B12 and folic acid. If you decide to drink coffee, take high levels of folic acid, vitamin B12, and biologicals with laboratory monitoring to make sure the treatment is appropriate. The homocysteine level should be at the lowest limit of normal because it is a toxic substance produced by the body during the metabolism of certain amino acids. It causes arterial obstruction and dementia, Parkinson's disease, and other brain disorders.

• **Effect on the central nervous system.** The central nervous system consists of the brain and spinal cord. The brain requires a large amount of energy to function properly and for its own development. It also requires an increased amount of myelin (a fatty substance that insulates nerve cells) as it forms an increased number of synapses (the space between nerve cells through which one nerve cell communicates with the next by emitting neurotransmitters, including dopamine and acetylcholine), thereby improving neuronal communication within the brain. An adequate amount of T3 is also necessary for the brain to use glucose for energy. That's how T3, together with other hormones (DHEA, pregnenolone, testosterone, progesterone, and estradiol) contribute to our ability to think, to remember, to process information, and to concentrate.

T3 is especially important for brain development in the fetus, as well as in infants and young children.

A lack of thyroid hormones and other hormones can cause concentration difficulties and lead to depression and various neurological diseases, including Alzheimer's disease, Parkinson's disease, dementia, ADHD, autism, panic attacks (as a result of an increase in the level of serotonin in the brain), confusion, brain fog, and hearing noises or voices in the brain. A lack of thyroid hormones can also result in psychiatric disorders such as hallucinations, delusions, mania, schizophrenia (see the case report in Chapter 6), bipolar disorder, personality disorders, and compulsive thoughts, as well as addiction to alcohol, smoking, or food; tantrums; postpartum depression; bad dreams; and suicide. The treatment should start as early as possible and should be accompanied by a balance of other hormones that work in the brain. The diagnostic problem arises when doctors rely solely on the results of a TSH test.

• **Effect on bones:** Working in concert with other hormones and vitamin K2, T3 stimulates and balances bone production, growth, and mechanisms of structural design. T3 stimulates the growth of healthy bones at any age, especially during childhood when there is increased growth. An optimal level of the T3 hormone maintains the fluids inside the joints, preventing cartilage wear and pain, knee problems, joint wear and tear, and osteoporosis. All of these complaints may be a signal of a decreased output of thyroid hormones and other hormones.

• **Effect on muscle activity:** Together with testosterone and IGF-1, T3 has an effect on muscle building and muscle breakdown (anabolism and catabolism). T3 mobilizes whole proteins that will strengthen the muscle. An optimal amount of the hormone in the body will result in proper muscle functioning—that is, flexibility, strength, and endurance. In old age, we need optimal levels of these three hormones to maintain the appropriate structure of skeletal muscles; otherwise, we weaken because of muscle weakness. Overtraining increases cortisol levels and reduces the T3 level (see case report in Chapter 6).

• **Effect on skin:** A low level of T3 reduces blood flow to the skin. That's why you may experience dry skin, hair loss, an itchy scalp, psoriasis, dandruff, cracks in the feet, eczema, impetigo, slow wound healing, chronic itching, vitiligo, various skin allergies, and cold hands and feet. The nails are also damaged. The root of the nail lowers its activity because low T3,

• **Effect on the immune system.** Diseases related to the dysfunction of the immune system may arise. Hypothyroidism has been found in individuals with many conditions, some of which are autoimmune, such as celiac disease, type 1 and 2 diabetes, insulin resistance, Addison's disease, Cushing's disease, Sjogren's disease, ovarian failure or insufficiency, chronic fatigue syndrome, rheumatic arthritis, systemic lupus erythematosus (SLE), multiple sclerosis, sarcoidosis, and scleroderma. Achieving optimal levels of T3 can help resolve or alleviate these diseases. We will discuss this subject further in Chapter 7. A T3 test, according to the criteria I have established, can be used to help diagnose and treat these diseases (see below).

• **Tics and sensory disturbances:** The constant movement of legs, arms, hands, back, and face can be triggered in children and adults by a low temperature and a low level of T3. Doctors do not detect these problems when they rely solely on the results of a TSH test. A low level of T3 in the brain can trigger an overreaction in a specific area of the brain that may cause the individual to move. It may also trigger body movement in children with ADHD.

• **Pain:** T3 plays a role in minimizing migraine, chronic headaches, back pain, wrist pain, joint pain, carpal tunnel disease, foot tunnel disease, stiff joints, tendinitis, foot spurs, muscle spasms, muscle and bone pain, pain in the jaw (temporomandibular joint pain), chronic pain syndrome, and fibromyalgia (see Chapter 10).

• **Eyes:** You may complain of focusing problems, double vision, dry eyes, sensation of sand in the eyes, blurred vision, drooping eyelids, sensitivity to light, eyelid tics, red eyes due to inflammation, problems with night vision (due to low vitamin A also, and a dark ring around the eyes. Swelling and edema may be seen under the eyes, and the patient may exhibit symptoms of glaucoma or cataracts.

• **Ears:** A lack of T3 may result in hypersensitivity to noise, ringing in the ears, hearing loss, tinnitus, pain in the ears, a large amount of earwax, dizziness and vertigo.

• **Mouth and throat:** A lack of T3 may contribute to the development of swallowing disorders, the sensation of a lump or foreign object in the throat, pain in the neck, goiter, a swollen tongue, a sensation of suffocating, disturbances in the sense of taste, a craving for salty or sweet foods, speech problems, dry mouth, an unpleasant smell from the mouth, a tendency to develop caries, a low and hoarse voice, and bleeding or swelling of the gums.

• **Menstrual disorders:** Women develop many symptoms as a result of a low level of T3 because of the close interactions between the hormones of the thyroid gland and the ovaries. These symptoms include the cessation of menstruation, weak or heavy menstruation, irregular menstruation, short or very long menstruation, severe pain during menstruation, failure to ovulate, permanent or persistent vaginal bleeding, pain before or during menses (premenstrual syndrome [PMS]), mood swings before or during menstruation (premenstrual tension), water and gas retention during menstruation, signs of late or early puberty, menstrual disorders during the first few months of puberty, early or late menopause, difficult menopause, endometriosis, polycystic ovaries, and polycystic breasts. We will discuss these in Chapter 8.

• **Fertility or pregnancy disorders:** These problems also arise in part because of the interconnection of functions of hormones of the thyroid gland and the ovaries. These problems include infertility, miscarriage, stillbirths, and in vitro fertilization failures; abnormal levels of estradiol, progesterone, or testosterone; reduced secretion of vaginal fluid, resulting in vaginal dryness and pain during intercourse; abnormal sperm or a low sperm count; decreased libido; polycystic breasts; anemia, diabetes, or high blood pressure during pregnancy; placental abruption; heavy bleeding after birth or a prolonged birth process due lack of expansion of the cervix; slow scar healing and pain around surgical scars; inadequate milk production; premature birth or abnormal (high or low) birthweight; and evidence of a lack of development or prolonged jaundice, autism, ADD/ADHD, or malformations. These will be discussed in Chapter 9.

• **Emotional problems:** Inadequate T3 levels can contribute to stress, mental restlessness, the desire to be alone, mood swings, anxiety, a personality change, feeling insulted, restlessness, being easily startled, mistrust, fear, and excessive excitability (see case report in Chapter 6).

• **Kidneys and urinary bladder:** Inadequate T3 levels can contribute to a lack of control over urine flow, particularly during sleep; chronic inflammation of the bladder; the formation of stones in the kidneys and gallbladder; recurrent infections of the urinary tract; and kidney failure.

• **Lungs:** Inadequate T3 availability in the respiratory tract can result in asthma, bronchitis, emphysema, breathing difficulties, pleural effusion, shortness of breath, and pneumonia.

• **Cancer:** An inadequate amount of T3 and T4 and an increased amount of rT3 have been associated with all types of cancer, including cancer of the skin; thyroid, prostate, and other glands; lungs; and breast.

• **Endocrine (hormone-secreting) glands:** Because T3 is necessary for the production of energy and heat in the cells of every gland, it is essential for the production of every type of hormone. If the amount of T3 that is produced is inadequate, the other glands will exhibit signs of a reduction in their hormone secretions. The glands that are most likely to be affected before age 40 are the adrenals, ovaries, testicles, and pituitary gland, as well as the thyroid gland itself.

It may seem unbelievable that so many symptoms can appear due to a decrease in body temperature and energy production. I couldn't believe it at first, either. But when I heard the complaints from my patients, I understood the importance of this hormone. Many complaints are about mild symptoms that most people can deal with. Some, however, are severe and significantly disrupt the quality of life. These are complaints that patients tell the attending physician or specialist, who usually does not see the overall picture and relies mainly on the results of blood tests (the appearance of a red asterisk) or other tests to verify your condition then uses drugs or surgery to treat the symptoms without treating the cause of the disease. The correct method for decoding the lab test can help us understand what is going on.

Frequently hypothyroidism is accompanied by other hormonal disorders. You may be forced to continue living with your complaints for years or turn to alternative medicine or look for another professional to soothe your complaints. If the cause and root of the problem are not treated at the beginning, you may develop irreversible physical changes that reduce your quality of life for years to come.

How It Started

Once we have all the data, I can assess how this phenomenon of a low T3 level develops. In most cases, it starts at a young age (before age 30 years), depending on the person's lifespan. At that age, the T3 level in the blood is at its best—in the upper third of the normal range. Over the years, for many reasons (including stress, an inadequate diet, and alcohol), the T3 level decreases. You may recall that consuming carbohydrates before bed lowers the production of important hormones in the pituitary gland, including TSH. Other factors that may reduce hormone production in the pituitary include an increase of cortisol, which reduces 5'D activity, which, in turn, reduces the T3 output. There could also be a high level of rT3, which prevents T3 from entering the cell. In any case, the T3 level inside the cells becomes insufficient to generate enough energy and heat. Whatever the reason, the patient begins to complain about various symptoms (such as menstrual disorders or fatigue) indicating that the body is not functioning correctly due to a lack of energy. In general, these complaints are treated symptomatically. The treatment offered by practitioners of functional medicine is based on the blood test results for all of the main hormones to see which one is not present in an adequate amount (Table 4-1). If the level of T3 or any other hormones that should have a reading in the central part of the normal average range is low, it means that the T4/T3 conversion rate in the liver is abnormal or there is a low level of progesterone, testosterone, and other hormones, as well as several vitamins (including vitamin E) and minerals (including selenium). The best result is when T3 and other essential hormone levels are close to the upper normal average range.(Table 4-1)

Lab Checklist

In addition to a blood count and general tests, the following lab tests are necessary to make an accurate diagnosis of disease: TSH, FT3, FT4, estradiol and progesterone (in women), cortisol (at 8 am), anti-thyroid peroxidase antigen (TPO Ag), insulin-like growth factor-1 (IGF-1), dehydroepiandrosterone (DHEA), testosterone (in men), iron, ferritin, vitamin D, and vitamin B12.

Treatment

The proprietary names of the T4 hormone supplements are Eltroxin®, Euthyroid, and Synthroid®. Each tablet contains 50 micrograms of natural or biological hormone. T3 is also manufactured under many names; those that appear on the internet include Tyromel® and Cytomel®. T3 can also be obtained at HMOs under its generic name: T3-iodothyronine sodium. Each tablet contains 25 micrograms of T3. Natural hormones are destroyed in the stomach or during digestion or not absorbed well, particularly if you have digestive absorption problems. Thus, it is better to put the tablet behind the upper lip (if you want to eat) or under the tongue and wait until it melts so it can be absorbed slowly into the oral mucosa. Monitor your temperature once a day while lying in bed before rising then again about an hour after lunch until you feel well again. By then, your body temperature will have risen to about 37 degrees and will have remained there throughout the day, or your T3 level will have reached the upper third of its normal upper limit.

If your doctor starts with 50 micrograms of T4, don't take more, because it may convert to rT3 instead of the active T3 and block the entry of T3 into the cell. Put the pill under your tongue or behind your upper lip every morning so it can be absorbed slowly. This method has several advantages:
• It avoids rapid absorption of T3, which, in sensitive or anxious people, can produce a fast pulse, shortness of breath, and other unpleasant feelings. These feelings will overpass after a while, however

- It allows you to eat immediately, provided you put the tablet under your upper lip and don't swallow it
- It bypasses the digestive system, because often the hormone is not fully absorbed. You have to take a supplement to improve 5'D activity and T4/T3 conversion.

After the age of 50, before starting this treatment, you should rule out heart disease, blockage of arteries in the neck, cancer, and other diseases through an ultrasound examination of the abdomen, prostate, female reproductive system, and other parts of the body. This has to be done, because when an adverse event occurs during treatment, the doctor and the patient will attribute this event to the new, unknown treatment with natural hormones and not to the patient's previous condition. That's why I prefer to give the patient an accepted treatment using T4 with 5'D supplemental support to increase the conversion of T4 to T3 while monitoring the patient's temperature. It is possible to continue treatment with the drug at a lower dose. Recently I started giving T3 alone in small doses to avoid problems with the T4/T3 conversion.

The appearance of a new disease during treatment has nothing to do with hormonal replacement treatment, because the natural approach has no side effects and does not cause new diseases like drugs do. If the patient's body temperature doesn't rise, you need to find out why: Is it because of a low conversion rate; poor absorption; selenium, iron and other mineral deficiency; a high rT3 level; or cooking with PUFA oils (these, which include canola oil, are liquid at room temperature but do not include olive oil), which may contribute to T3 resistance by competing with T3 to gain entry into body cells? If so, you may start treatment with T3, taking half a tablet (12.5 micrograms) every 7 to 10 days and increasing the dosage slowly until the body temperature reaches 36.8 to 37 degrees each day. The maximum dose is 50 micrograms per day. Once the patient can take the maximum dose, it should be taken as 25 micrograms twice a day—once in the morning and once at mid-day. If T3 is taken later in the day, the T3 level in the morning may be high and give your doctor the impression that you have hyperthyroidism. I recently started using desiccated thyroid gland from ruminated cows that contains T4 and T3. The rise in temperature is a long process, one that may take a month after all the enzymatic systems are activated. When the patient reports that his physical condition has improved and his body temperature has remained stable, it may be a sign that the appropriate dose has been found. If the T3 level is below the upper limit of normal, I recommend a natural diet without trans fats x or reduced as possible to ensure the proper entry of T3 into the cells.

In general, the T4/T3 conversion process is very good in children and adolescents. They can achieve the desired body temperature by taking T4 25 micrograms per day. For normal 5'D activity, the patient will need vitamins A and D, as well as selenium, iron and progesterone. A T3 dose of 25 micrograms twice a day for 3 months will improve enzymatic activity within the mitochondria so that you can utilize glucose and cholesterol better. By monitoring the body temperature, one can treat a morbid phenomenon at an early stage. As the body heat increases, the complaints gradually decrease. The patient usually informs me that his energy level has improved and that he is even losing some weight.

A nutritious diet is also necessary to improve 5'D enzyme activity in the mitochondria. Healthy food, 8 to 9 hours of sleep, a protein diet (especially before sleep), and the elimination of allergies can change your life for the better. Other hormonal supplements may be necessary, however. If so, take them under medical supervision based on blood test results, as needed.

Hashimoto's disease—when the body attacks the thyroid gland

Hashimoto's disease, which was first described by a Japanese researcher of the same name, is an autoimmune disease in which the patient produces antibodies against the thyroid enzymes thyroid peroxidase (TPO) and the colloidal media protein thyroglobulin (TG). This condition is also called chronic inflammation of the thyroid gland. It is diagnosed after a swelling appears in the area of the thyroid gland in the neck. It is accompanied by digestive disorders and symptoms of hypothyroidism. Hashimoto's disease is detected using a blood test for antibodies against each of these two mediums. This is the most common autoimmune disease. Various factors can cause its development. Eventually the gland function will be damaged, along with its ability to produce its hormones. As a result, the TSH hormone level rises.

When Hashimoto's disease is suspected, the entire hormonal system should be tested. There should also be tests for antibodies against TPO and TG antigens (Ag), as well as such viruses as Epstein-Barre virus (EPV), cytomegalovirus (CMV), and COVID-19; antigens against these infections may also appear in individuals with other autoimmune diseases, including type 1 diabetes, systemic lupus erythematosus [SLE], or lupus), and arthritis. The reasons why the immune system produces antibodies that attack the gland are multifaceted, but the level of antibodies should be zero if the immune system does not attack the gland. The appearance of antibodies alone is enough to diagnose the disease. And don't wait for a red star!

Hashimoto's disease is frequently characterized by hypothyroidism in women because of their high estradiol levels. In this situation, the liver cannot break down estradiol; instead, it is excreted through the urine but reabsorbed from the feces. Estradiol metabolites accumulate in the blood and damage the gland.

Another possible cause of hypothyroidism involves its vulnerability to free radicals on its structure. Free radicals are oxygen atoms that contain an unpaired electron, which makes them electrically unstable. This instability allows them to bond with any substance in the cell—including fats, proteins, and DNA—and change its atomic structure. Once the atomic structure is changed, the function of that structure in body organs is cancelled. This type of tissue damage can trigger human disease.

The body protects tissue from such damage by producing enzymes called antioxidants (such as glutathione and superoxide dismutases [SODs]), which can neutralize free radicals immediately. When the number of free radicals overwhelms the number of antioxidants, however, the body is at risk for disease. This risk is increased when the body does not have enough of the mineral selenium (which antioxidants need to function efficiently) or the supplement N-acetyl cysteine (or NAC). In individuals with Hashimoto's disease, the number of free radicals on the surface of the thyroid gland is increased and selenium levels are low. The resulting damage to the thyroid gland by the free radicals reduces its activity and results in hypothyroidism.

How antioxidants reduce free radicals

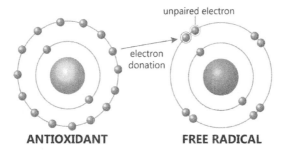

Figure 5-5. Interaction between free radicals and antioxidants.

Free radicals attach to the TPO enzyme or the TG protein, thereby changing their three-dimensional atomic shape and compromising their ability to function. The change in the structure of TPO and TG is not so extensive that the immune system cannot recognize them; and when it does, it attacks the thyroid gland and damages it, causing it to produce fewer T4 and T3 hormones.

1. The immune system reacts by producing more antibodies against the thyroid gland. Many women with menstrual disturbances develop Hashimoto's disease. It is 20 times more common in women than in men, because women produce significantly more estradiol than men.

2. Because of high estradiol levels, the body is exhausted by stress, which raises the cortisol level, which, in turn, affects 5'D activity.

3. In people who are sensitive to gluten, Hashimoto's disease begins with gastrointestinal complaints and symptoms of menstrual disturbances. Gluten can cause a local inflammation in the mucous layer lining the small intestine. This layer consists of a single layer of cells. An overgrowth of harmful bacteria and Candida organisms (fungi) results in the production of toxins that can damage the integrity of the mucosal layer. This is especially common in people with a low level of the antibody immunoglobulin A (IgA). This is a common finding in patients with autoimmune disease and in families suffering from recurrent respiratory tract infections such as chronic sinusitis and celiac disease. Microscopic passageways form between mucus cells in the intestine and may reach the bloodstream (Figure 5-6). Thus, pathogens can circulate throughout the body and settle in any tissue in the body (leaky bowel disease).

4. I have already mentioned that herpes viruses, cytomegalovirus, Epstein-Barre virus, and COVID-19 can also settle in

the thyroid gland, causing a local inflammation and an immune response.
Therefore, when there is a suspicion that a problem originates in the thyroid gland or involves its hormones, it is always advisable to check for the presence of antibodies against TPO, TG, and the viruses just mentioned to rule out a history of viral infection and check the Ig A level.

Inflammation can cause the thyroid gland to swell and trigger the formation of soft inflammatory structures consisting of many blood vessels and immune cells (mainly lymphocytes). A biopsy may be performed to rule out cancer.

Laboratory tests to detect Hashimoto's disease
The tests required to confirm the presence of Hashimoto's disease include tests for thyroid hormone levels (TSH, FT3, and FT4) and antibodies against thyroid enzymes (TPO and TG), as well as vitamin D, DHEA, parathyroid hormone (PTH), immunoglobulin A, iron (ferritin), zinc, and 8 am cortisol. Women of childbearing age should also be tested for LH, FSH, estradiol, and progesterone to rule out estradiol dominance syndrome. Their tests should be made on days 18 to 24 of the menstrual cycle. Testosterone should also be tested in men.

Symptom complaints
In most cases, patients complain about symptoms of hypothyroidism and estradiol hormone overcontrol, including fatigue, lack of sleep, anxiety, water retention, muscle spasms, and heavy menstruation with blood clots. The physician should ask for a platelets blood test (especially if the patient is using an anti-conception pill to control menstrual bleeding), because a high number of platelets predisposes the woman to the forma-

tion of vein clots, which puts her at risk for sudden death due to a lung embolism. There is an acute change in blood sugar levels, increase in carbohydrates consumption, and hypertension. Their blood tests may show low levels of magnesium and iron, as well as T3, T4, progesterone, and vitamin D; and a high level of cortisol, C-reactive protein, and estradiol.

Treatment of Hashimoto's disease

1. The treatment of Hashimoto's disease is based on several principles:
2. Regulation of the bacterial population in the digestive system.
3. Abolition of gluten intake.
4. Regulation of the level of estradiol and other hormones, including progesterone (please see the next section).
5. Avoidance of environmental toxins, including perfumes and creams containing estradiol-like substances and foods.
6. Hormonal treatment of the thyroid gland with only T3, which can trigger avoid the T4 conversion problems.
7. Hormonal balance of other glands, if necessary.
8. Improvement in the function of the 5'D enzyme and glutathione. Multivitamins, zinc, magnesium, and calcium supplements may be helpful.
9. Self-study of the disease.
10. Treatment with minerals and vitamins.
11. Anti-aromatase supplement to reduce the estradiol level.

Actually, the first step in the treatment of Hashimoto's disease is to lower the level of estradiol. This hormone damages the gland's structure and lowers its activity and rate of metabolism throughout the body. As a result, the liver becomes overloaded trying to filter out increasing levels of estradiol metabolites, which can further damage the thyroid gland and promote cancer. To prevent this, I use a progesterone ointment that provides 20 to 40 milligrams of progesterone cream twice a day (see Chapter 8), as well as vitamins A, D, and E; the B vitamins; selenium (to support 5'D activity); and a gluten-free diet (to reduce the number of antibodies). A high-protein diet during the day (see Chapter 8) and sometimes meditation can be helpful to reduce stress and cortisol levels and strengthen the immune system.

Case report: A patient with Hashimoto's disease

Test Name	Results	Units	Reference Values	Normal Range
TSH	0.76	uIU/L	0.4-4.2	.......*............
Free T4	17	pmol/L	10-20	................*...
Free T3	3.6	pmol/L	3.5-6.5	..*...............
Thyroglobulin	more 20	kIU/L	0-50	.........*......
Anti TPO AG's	19.5	kIU/L	0-35	.........*.......

Figure 5-7. A 34-year-old patient with Hashimoto's disease with high Thyroglobulin and Thyroid peroxid antibodies was treated with 100 milligrams of T4. The FT4 is over the center of the normal range, reflecting the high T4 dose. The FT3 level is very low, however. The reason for the patient's complaints, therefore, may be a defect in the conversion of T4 to T3 because the inflammation and a block enter of T3 into the cells because the high rT3.

Graves' Disease, or Hyperthyroidism

Sometimes the thyroid gland is damaged by an autoimmune disease, but the immune system continues to produce special antibodies. For instance, instead of destroying the TPO enzyme, it activates this enzyme in a way similar to that of the TSH hormone. As a result, hyperactivity of the thyroid gland—Graves' disease—develops. The background to this disease consists of the same factors that cause hypothyroidism in Hashimoto's disease, but the antibodies target TSH receptors on the surface of the gland and activate the TPO enzyme to oversecrete the T4 and T3 hormones. As a result, the gland grows and its hormonal activity and metabolic rate increase throughout the whole body. Graves' disease is more common in women than in men. It appears at all ages, but with a much lower frequency than Hashimoto's disease.

What are the symptoms of high T3 levels?

Because of the high metabolic rate in Graves' disease, its symptoms are the opposite of those of hypothyroidism: The body temperature increases, weight loss occurs (despite an increased appetite), and the skin becomes moist due to excessive sweating. Patients with this disorder also exhibit muscle wasting, fatigue and weakness, nervousness and emotional restlessness, increased bowel activity and diarrhea, an increased heart rate, and weak muscle pain. If the illness continues for a long time, the muscles and tissues in the eye socket become depleted and the patient exhibits protrusion of the eyes.

Laboratory tests

The TSH asterisk is red and below normal, and the FT3 and FT4 asterisks are red and above the upper limit of normal. Blood tests are positive for the anti-TPO antigen or anti-TSH antigen. A relevant case is described following the section on treatment.

Treatment of Graves' disease

The accepted conventional treatment for Graves' disease consists of drugs such as mercaptizol (methimazole) to reduce the production of thyroid gland hormones. Some people cannot continue this treatment, however, because of nausea, vomiting, skin rashes, headaches, hair loss, muscle pain, and other complaints. To slow down the heart rate, people are given drugs called beta blockers. Some naturopaths recommend nutritional supplements such as bugleweed, gypsiorthid, club moas, or lemon balm and rishi, shiitake, or maitake mushrooms. These are supposed to block TSH receptors and stabilize the T3 level. I have no experience with these plants. In most cases, patients are treated with radioactive iodine or surgery to remove part of the gland. So it is easier to improve their condition with T3, as I explained in the previous chapter.

Patients should maintain the same rules regarding diet, nutritional supplements, physical activity, etc., as described in the section on underactivity of the thyroid gland resulting from Hashimoto's disease.

Case report: A 30-year-old woman with signs of hyperthyroidism

A 30-year-old woman with clinical and laboratory signs of hyperthyroidism was treated with Japanese mushrooms.

Thyroid Hormone	Value	Unit of Measure	Normal Range
TSH 0.01		mIU/L	0.55 – 4.78
FT3	18.3	pmol/L	3.5-6.5
FT4	50.2	pmol/L	10-20

Figure 5-8a. Thyroid hormone test results for the 30-year-old female patient. The measurements in red indicate hyperthyroidism. This information was taken from Facebook.

Thyroid Hormone	'Value	Unit of Measure	Normal Range
TSH	10.67	mIU/L	0.55-4.78
FT3	4.22	pmol/L	3.5-6.5
FT4	10.67	pmol/L	10-20

Figure 5-8b. Thyroid hormone test results following treatment with Japanese mushrooms. There was also an improvement in symptoms. Note the low FT3 value and high TSH value. This means that she was still having some symptoms of hypothyroidism. I referred her to the naturalist to arrange her treatment.

Chapter 6

Presentation of Cases and Correct Diagnosis of Thyroid Disease

Suppose you have already had blood tests for all the thyroid hormones. In that case, it is important that you know how to correctly interpret the results. I have described an approach that enables an accurate diagnosis of the diseases mentioned in this book.

The important thing in making a diagnosis is to notice where the asterisk is located within the range of average values. The absolute numbers are unimportant, because each laboratory uses a different test method; therefore, the normal values frequently vary from laboratory to laboratory. Remember that when we are young, our T3 values are in the upper third of the normal range. As a result, the body temperature is 37 degrees Celsius most of the day; this allows us to run about and be energetic (Figure 6-1). Over the years, the asterisk will change its position to opposite values. When it reaches a point at which its level in the blood is not sufficient to get to all the cells in the body, we feel something—usually fatigue, or perhaps another complaint. At this point, the doctor might say that the test result is normal because the asterisk appears within the normal range compared with the general population. Over the years, or as a result of some acute event, the T3 asterisk moves to an even lower range, reaching the lower third of the normal range (Figure 6-2). At that point, any disease may appear because, overall, the body is not functioning well due to a "lack of energy production." Therefore, it is more important to pay attention to the position of the asterisk for T3 (or any other hormone) within its normal range and compare the result with its position in individuals aged 20 to 40 30 years old (Table 6-1). Then you will find the reason for your complaint. Any change in the position of the asterisk position toward the "wrong" direction will cause complaints that intensify as the asterisk reaches the other side of the curve, even before the appearance of a red asterisk. To remind you of the normal location of thyroid hormones, I have provided a chart showing the asterisk within a graphic representation of its normal range in blood tests (Figure Table 6-1).

Name	Results	Normal Range
TSH	lower than 2 mIU/L	0.4(.. *...........)4.2
Free T4	15 pmol/L	10(......*.......)20
Free T3	5.8 pmol/L	3.5(..........*...)6.5

Table 6-1. A normal range for each of the thyroid hormones. Abbreviations: TSH, thyroid-stimulating hormone; FT4, free thyroxine (T4); FT3, free triiodothyronine (T3).

Case 1: Patient with hypothyroidism based on a TSH test and after testing FT4 and FT3

This patient presents some typical dilemmas. There are situations in which the blood test results are "seemingly" normal because they fall within the normal range, but the T3 level is not sufficient for the normal functioning of the body. Figure 6-2 shows the blood test results taken while the patient complained of weight gain, hair loss, chronic fatigue, mood changes, and muscle pain, and a body temperature of 36.5 degrees Celsius.

Test Name	Results	Units	Reference Values	Normal Range
FT4	1.27	ng/dL	0.70-1.80	........*....
FT3	109.17	ng/dL	80-200	...*........
TSH	3.1	mIU/dL	0.2-5.00	........*..

Figure 6-2. Results of thyroid hormone tests for a 53-year-old woman with complaints of weakness, low body temperature, and fibromyalgia. All the values are within the "normal range," but the patient's complaints suggest "low T3 syndrome." The test findings supporting this diagnosis are as follows: the T3 value is at the lower limit of the normal range; the TSH reading is above 2, and the FT4 value is in the middle range (as it should be if the thyroid gland is producing enough T4). There are signs of a disturbance in the conversion of T4 to T3, however, and the TSH value is above 2 because the hypothalamus reacts to a low T3 level and low body temperature.

Case 2: Effect of a serious illness on the activity of the thyroid gland

This is the case of a 70-year-old man with cancer. He is receiving oncological treatment that is affecting his 5'D enzyme activity (Figure 6-3). [Many other serious diseases show the same picture in laboratory tests.] It is possible that the cancer is related to the fact that a low level of T3 weakens the immune system, thereby leaving the body unprotected against many diseases.

125

Test Name	Results	Normal Range	Units
Thyroxine T4 Free Blood	1.12	0.17(...*........)-2.0	ng/dl
Free T3 Blood	32.38	*80(..............)200	ng/dl
TSH Blood	1.58	0.40(....*........)4.7	mIU/L

Figure 6-3. Thyroid test results for a 70-year-old patient being treated for rectal cancer. The T3 level is below normal because the patient's oncology treatment has damaged the activity of the 5'D enzyme. TSH alone is not an indicator of a lack of energy production.

Case 3: Patient with a head injury

A young man was seen after a road accident, during he which he experienced a head injury. As a result of this injury, the pituitary gland stopped secreting TSH, because the hypothalamus stopped secreting thyroid-releasing hormone (TRH) (see Figure 6-4). The thyroid gland also stopped producing T4 and T3 and heat and energy as well. Therefore, improvement in his condition and his rehabilitation will take a long time. To improve the situation, I recommended treatment with T4 and T3 hormones (Figure 6-4).

Test Name	Results	Normal Range	Units
Free T4	4.11	*7.........)17	pmp/L
Testosterone	19.27	(5.4....*...)28	nmol/L
Free T3	3.08	*3.8(........)6	pmp/L
TSH	0.08	*0.34(...........)5.6	mIU/L
HB(A1C)	5.08%	4.(.........*.)5.7	%

Figure 6-4. Results of thyroid and testosterone blood tests for a 34-year-old man following a car accident in which he experienced a head injury. The patient's complaints indicate severe hypothyroidism. The blood tests show that his pituitary gland is not producing TSH and hypothalamus dysfunction;

as a result, his T3 and T4 levels are very low. The production of testosterone has not been affected, however. Additionally, his hemoglobin A1C and blood glucose levels are high because the mitochondria are not using glucose to create energy in the presence of a low level of T3.

Case 5: Patient with a CMV viral infection

A 51-year-old woman with a history of high fever, swollen lymph nodes, laboratory tests that are positive for CMV, and high IgG antibody levels presented with a body temperature of 36 degrees. Since the acute phase of the illness passed, she has been complaining for several months about considerable weakness. The doctor measured her TSH level, which was 1.3 milli-international units per milliliter (mIU/L)—which is within normal limits. In a test taken by a private laboratory, her T3 and T4 levels indicated the cause of her complaints (Figure 6-5).

Test Name	Results	Normal Range	Units
Free T4 Vidas	0.95	(0.7...*.......)-2.0	ng/dl
Free T3 Vidas	2.81	(2.6..*........)5.04	pgt/ml
TSH Vidas		(0.3...........)5.0	uIU/ml

Figure 6-5. Blood test results for a 51-year-old woman with a history of a high body temperature, swollen lymph nodes, and tests that were positive for CMV and increased immunoglobulin G (IgG) antibodies. Her blood test results indicate that her FT4 level must be 1.35 (0.7 + 2.0 = 2.7 ÷ 2 = 1.35), but it is below the mid-normal range. That means her thyroid gland is producing less T4 hormone, probably due to the viral infection in the thyroid gland. A low-normal FT3 level explains her fatigue. The optimal level is near 5.40. She received T3 hormone treatment, which improved her condition considerably. A similar phenomenon occurs in other viral diseases.

Case 6: A 55-year-old woman with menopausal complaints and high cholesterol.

Name	Value	Units	Reference value	Range
TSH	2.49	mIU/L	0.3-4.2	….......*…
FT4	13.8	pmol/L	10-20.0	…..*…...
FT3	3.8	pmol/L	3.5-6.5	.*………
CHOLESTEROL	250.5	mg/dL	110-200	………..*
CHOLESTEROL HDL	79	mg/dL	40.-120	…...*…...
CHOLESTEROL LDL	155.1	mg/dL	40-130	…..……..*
NON HDL CHOLESTEROL	172	mg/dL	35-150	………..*
DHEA-S	1.95	mmol/L	0.9-11.6	..*………

Figure 6.6. Results of blood tests for a 55-year-old woman with complaints of weakness, low body temperature, and signs of menopause. In most of the results, the asterisk is within the "normal range." Consequently, she was diagnosed with hypothyroidism. Note that the T3 asterisk is within the lower limit of normal, the TSH reading is above 2, and the FT4 result is in the middle range (as it should be, given that the thyroid is producing enough T4). There are signs of a disturbance in the conversion of T4 to T3, however: The TSH value is above 2 and the T3 level is low, as is the body temperature. The total cholesterol and LDL levels are high due to hypothyroidism. She is also under a mild amount of stress, as indicated by her cortisol level, which is not in the lower third of average values. Her testosterone and DHEA results are low, as can be the case in menopausal women.

After treatment with 25 micrograms of T3, progesterone 20 mg twice a day, a very low dose of estradiol gel (1.25 g Oestrogel) once a day, and a multivitamin supplement, she feels better, and this is reflected in her lab results (Figure 6-7).

Name	Value	Units	Reference value	Range
TSH	2.02	mIU/L	0.6-4.8	.*..........
FT4	16	pmol/L	10-20.0	.......*...
FT3	4.6	pmol/L	3.5-6.5	....*........
CHOLESTEROL	158.2	mg/dL	110-200	.........*....
CHOLESTEROL HDL	54	mg/dL	40.-120	..*.........
CHOLESTEROL LDL	89.1	mg/dL	40-130	...*..........
NON HDL CHOLESTEROL	105	mg/dL	35-150	........*.....

Figure 6-7. The lab results obtained for the previous 55-year-old woman one month after she started treatment for symptoms of menopause and hypothyroidism . Her TSH values are normal, her FT4 level is in the correct range, and her FT3 level increased slightly. She is now taking T3 50 micrograms daily. Her cholesterol level is normal, but her progesterone and estradiol levels have increased slightly. For this reason, I increased the dose of progesterone to 40 mg per day.

Case 7: Patient with a diagnosis of epilepsy

The wife of J.A., a 70-year-old man, called to tell me that her husband had an attack of epilepsy that caused him to fall backward and break three vertebrae. The medication he had received during his three hospitalizations had not helped. He was first given Depalept Chrono, which contains valproic acid and is often prescribed for various forms of epilepsy. He was then given the anticonvulsant drug, gabapentin. Unfortunately, gabapentin triggered an allergic reaction that consisted of diarrhea. skin scratching, and asthma. J.A. had a history of aortic stenosis and had received a biological aortic replacement valve. His coronary arteries were normal, but a brain MRI showed evidence of paracortical damage in the white matter, probably on a background of brain ischemia and marked by small vessel disease. He also has moderate renal failure, with a 50% reduction in renal function. The nephrologist recommended that he drink 1 liter of water daily. I requested a complete hormonal study (Figure 6-8).

Test			Patient Results	Reference Value
DHEA-S	µg/dL		237.4	80 - 560
TSH	µIU/mL		< 0.004	0.358 - 3.74
T4, Total	µg/dL		4.0	4.5 - 12.5
T3, Free	pg/mL		2.9	2.2 - 4.0
T4, Free	ng/dL		0.61	0.76 - 1.46
Cortisol	µg/dL		20.1	3.1 - 22.4
Anti-TPO Ab	IU/mL		< 10.0	0.0 - 35.0
Anti-Thyroglobulin Ab	IU/mL		< 20	ND - 40
Thyroglobulin	ng/mL		3.8	<= 55
Thyroxine-binding globulin, TBG	µg/mL		17.6	14 - 31
Reverse T3	ng/dL	[1]	12.2	9.0 - 27.0

Figure 6-8. The test results suggest the patient is in a stressful situation because the cortisol 8 am is high and the DHEA is low. The TSH is below normal due to the effect of anti-epileptic drugs on the hypothalamus. As a result, the FT4 and FT3 are low. The rT3 level is acceptable, however.

I first suggested that the patient seek the advice of a specialist to learn how to overcome his allergic reaction to the drugs using the NEAT approach. Because the MRI report suggested small-vessel disease in the brain and T3 dilates small vessels, I suggested T3 therapy, starting with 25 micrograms, while taking his body temperature two times a day (see Figure 6-9).

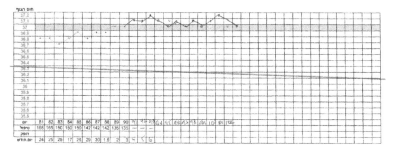

Figure 6-9. Body temperature for J.A. over 3 months of T3 therapy (50 micrograms/day).

I followed J.A. for 3 years. During that time, he did not have any seizures. I stopped his medications because his cholesterol and glucose levels were normal. He has been taking Q10 500 milligrams, T3 50 micrograms, testosterone 25 milligrams, and DHEA 25 milligrams daily (Figure 6-10).

Test Name	Results	Normal Range	Units	Range
Estradiol	90	less than 100	pmol/L	*(...............)
TSH	>0.009	0.3-5.0	mIU/dl	*(...............)
T3 Free	6.3	3.6-6.5	pmol/L	(..............*)
T4 Free	10.9	10-20.1	pmol/L	(*...............)
Testisterone	11.8	8-22.25	nmol/L	(......*...........)
IGF-1	25.75	3.8-36.5	nmol/L	(................*.....)
DHEA-S	1.37	1.42-11.0	pmol/L	*(................)
Cortisol	661	138-690	nmol/L	(............*)

Figure 6-10. Four months after starting treatment for seizures, J.A. was in distress because of a fear of having seizures after discontinuing his medications (as I suggested). One year later, he had a myocardial infarction caused by a severe obstruction of the left anterior descending artery. Before he was released from the hospital, the cardiologist recommended statins and anticoagulant drugs. J.A. asked him why he had a heart attack when his cholesterol and glucose levels were within their normal ranges and stated that he may continue

131

to take this medication. When he got home, he took the first dose of the statin and the anticoagulant drugs, but he had severe diarrhea and vomiting. When I visited him in his home, he was dehydrated and stopped during our conversation to vomit. I advised him to drink a lot of water. He did, and then he recovered. His lab test results appear in Figure 6-11.

Test Name	Results	Normal Range	Units	Range
Glucose	93	70-100	mg/dl	(.........*)
Urea	65.6	17-43	mg/dl	(.........)*
Creatinine	1.21	0.5-1.41	mg/dl	(.......*..)
Sodium	139.6	135-145	mEq/L	(..*........._
Potassium	4.5	3.5-5.1	mEq/L	(.....*.....)
Cholesterol	225	120*200	mg/dl	(.........)*
Thyglicerids	94	less than 150	mg/dl	*(.........)
Cholesterol HDL	37	more than 40	mg/dl	(.........*)
Cholesterol LDL calc	188	less than 130	mg/dl	(.........)*
Non HDL Chol	198	more than 160	mg/dl	(..*.....)
AstP (GST) 30	30	30-31	IUL	(*.........)

Figure 6-11. Laboratory values for J.A., a 70-year-old patient with epilepsy. The urea and creatinine levels were high because of renal dysfunction and dehydration.

When his condition improved, J.A. asked me why he had a heart attack if his cholesterol and blood sugar levels were normal. I told him there may have been another cause of the heart attack and recommended a homocysteine blood test (Figure 6-12).

Cardiac Markers	Results	Units	Range
Homocystine	31.8	umol/L	.(..........)*

Figure 6-12. Homocysteine lab results for J.A., a 70-year-old man with epilepsy. His homocysteine level is high.

132

I explained previously that homocysteine is a toxic substance that is produced by the body. It could damage the endothelial cells, which line the internal surface of the arteries, if the amount of nitric oxide they secreted were reduced (Figure 5-1) and his vitamin B12 and B6 and folic acid levels fell. I then discovered that drinking more than three cups of coffee reduced the level of these vitamins in the body. I prescribed the supplements Homocysteine Resist and Nitric Oxide Boost to reduce the level of this toxic substance in his body (Figure 6-12). He later complained of palpitations (Figure 6-13). I requested an echocardiographic study, which caught an irregular atrial fibrillation event of 78 beats per minute. This study revealed signs of heart failure, a 20% reduction in heart function, and enlargement of the left ventricle and atrium of the heart. I thought that his heart needed more energy to improve its left ventricular function and possibly reduce the size of the left atrium. I recommended a diuretic and T3 25 milligrams three times a day (T3 only works for several hours during the day). His complaints about palpitations stopped. This improvement can be seen in his electrocardiogram (ECG) (Figure 6-14).

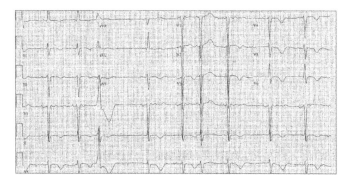

Figure 6-13. J.A.'s ECG shows atrial fibrillation and ventricular premature beats originating in the anterior wall of ventricle. It also shows evidence of a myocardial infarction in the anterior wall.

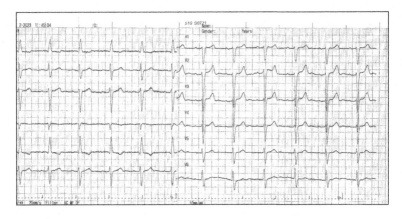

Figure 6-14. J.A.'s ECG shows a regular heart rhythm after treatment with T3 at 75 micrograms.

I learned a lot of new things with this patient.

Case 8: A patient with schizophrenia and obesity

A woman called to inform me that her 20-year-old obese son, who was being treated by a psychiatrist for schizophrenia, had not responded to treatment recently. I agreed to study the problem on the condition that the attending physician accepted my approach. After a short conversation, he accepted, and the hormonal tests were performed (Figures 6-15 to 6-17). During my conversation with the mother, I learned that he was a nice, quiet boy when he was a child, but another boy at school beat him badly several times and that during a vacation, he almost drowned, was saved but having swallowed a lot of sea water. Since then, he has been very aggressive. He broke the front door and a window in the office of the treating doctor.

Test Name	Results	Reference Values	Units	Range
TSH	4.61	0.55-4.78	uIU/L	(...............*)
Free T4	12.11	10.7-18.4	pg/dl	(..*.............)
Free T3	4.92	4.7-5.2	pg/dl	(..*...........)
FSH	0.74	0.95-11.95	uIU/mL	*(............)
LH	2.68	0.57-12.07	uIU/mL	(.....*..........)
Dhea-S	4.6	2.5-13.9	umol/	(.....*..........)
Testosterone	10.68	8.33-30.9	nmol/L	(.....*...........)
Cortisol	320	138-690	nmol/L	(.........*....)
IGF-1	169	117-323	ng/ml	(..*...........)

Figure 6-15. Lab report for a patient with schizophrenia and obesity revealed severe hypothyroidism. His FT3 and FT4 levels were very low, and his TSH level was high. His DHEA, testosterone, and IGF-1 levels were also low, suggesting that the mitochondria in the brain were not active at all. Because four hormones necessary for the normal functioning of the brain were at low levels, the FSH and LH were also low. I suspected treatment-related central hypogonadism. I then searched the literature for the effect of these anti-psychotic drugs on the hypothalamus.

I recommended that the attending physician reduce the dose for the psychiatric drugs, He explained to me that this patient has been very aggressive towards other people and had caused damage in his clinic. I explained to him that the resistance to psychiatric treatment was caused by his difficult hormonal situation. His mother did not agree to have her son transferred to a psychiatric hospital. I recommended that he start taking T3 12.5 milligrams and DHEA 25 milligrams daily. The doctor was very unsure because of the "side effects" of T3. I promised him that I would take responsibility for the treatment if he started with very low doses. The patient continued to take his medication. After a few months, his mother told me that he is quieter now and is at home. I suggested repeating the laboratory tests listed in Figure 6-15.

Test Name	Results	Reference Values	Units	Range
TSH	0.22	0.55-4.78	uIU/L	(.........*)
Free T4	8.66	10.7-18.4	pg/dl	*(...........)
Free T3	4.63	2.42-5.99	pg/dl	(..*...........)
Estradiol	59	40-161	pmol/L	(.........*.....)
FSH	0.8	0.95-11.95	uIU/mL	(....9...........)
LH	3.48	0.57-12.07	uIU/mL	*(............)
Dhea-S	16.8	2.5-13.9	umol/	(.....*..........)
Testosterone	6.77	9.33--3018	nmol/L	*(..............)
Cortisol	386.8	122-635.2	nmol/L	(.......*........)

Figure 6-16. After treatment with T3 50 micrograms daily and DHEA 50 milligrams daily, the patient's TSH and FT4 values were the same but his FT3 and the DHEA levels had increased. The testosterone, LH, and FSH levels were very low—did that reflect a hypothalamic-pituitary problem due to his antipsychotic drugs? There is a normal level for the patient to respond to replacement therapy with biological hormones. To improve the testosterone level, I suggested an anti-aromatase supplement and testosterone gel 25 milligrams to avoid an increase in estradiol caused by his obesity. His doctor accepted the recommendation to reduce the psychotic drugs because now he was absolutely quiet.

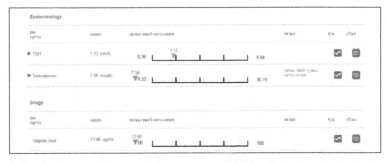

Figure 6-17. The patient's testosterone level was low despite the fact that his mother said she had been administering it to him herself. I increased the testosterone dose to 50 milligrams. She then sent me a long letter thanking me for the hormonal treatment that calmed her son and permitted him to return to his studies in the yeshiva.

Case 9: A patient being treated for overtraining

A 25-year-old professional boxer eats a carbohydrate-rich meal before he goes to bed and twice a day before he works out for at least one hour in the gym. He does so "to provide enough energy." He felt weak during a morning treatment session and was referred to the hospital for evaluation (Figure 6-18).

Name	Results	Units	References Values	Average Range
FT4	13.11	pmol/L	9.05-15.13	….........*…
FT3	4.85	pmol/L	2.42-5.99	….........*…
FSH	0.79	mIU/L	0.95-11.95	*…...........
LH	0.86	mIU/L	0.57-12.07	…*…....…...
TESTOSTERONE	2.57	nmpol/L	5.4-28	*…...........

Figure 6-18. During a morning training session, the patient, a 25-year-old prelesional boxer, felt considerably weak. A blood test showed abnormal thyroid gland activity due to an increase in FT4 and suboptimal FT3 levels during the training. Was there a disorder in the conversion of FT4 to FT3 due to a slightly elevated cortisol level? The attending endocrinologist made a diagnosis of central hypogonadism based on his low testosterone, FSH, and LH readings and recommended injections of gonadotropins to increase his LH and FSH levels. Other results were interpreted as normal, It is also a classic sign of the ability of high-carbohydrate evening meals to suppress nocturnal hormonal activity. The test showed that IGF-1 was at a level that would be considered optimal for a 25-year-old sportsman.

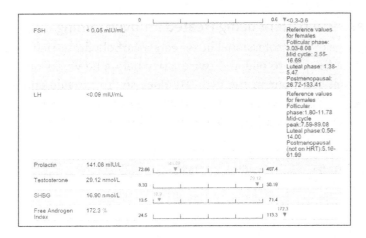

Figure 6-19. Test results after treatment with gonadotropins show an increase in testosterone. The SHIG level is low, as it should be, and the Free Androgen Index is high, which indicates the potential for very good sexual ability. The prolactin is normal.

His condition worsened as he was unable to lift weights or exercise in the gym due to severe weakness despite a normal testosterone level. The previous test revealed signs of thyroid hypoactivity due to a less-than-normal FT3, so I suggested a test of all of the thyroid hormones. The results appear in Figure 6-20.

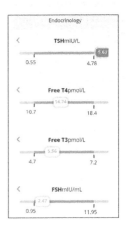

Figure 6-20. After stopping the treatment with gonadotropins, the patient's FSH level is still low. There are signs of hypothyroidism, however, given that he had an elevated TSH and a very low FT3 low due to problems converting T4 to T3. His FT4 level is good—almost in the center of the normal range. His body temperature was 36.1 degrees Celsius; during the middle of the day, it rose slightly to 36.5 degrees. I asked for general check-ins before he went to Dubai for a competition.

Uric Acid	7.19 mg/dL	3.5					7.2	
eGFR	>60 eGFR IU							eGFR IU = mL/min/1.73m מחושב לפי הנוסחה IDMSTraceable MDRD הנוסחה אינה מתאימה לשימוש עבור נשים בהריון, חולי דיאליזה ובמצבים של אי-ספיקת כליות חדה
LDH	340 U/L	0				▼		480
Creatine Kinase	175 U/L	0					171 ▼	175
AST(GOT)	26 U/L	0			▼		50	
ALT(GPT)	23 U/L	0			▼		50	
Alkaline Phosph.	67 U/L	30		▼			120	
Bilirubin, Total	0.95 mg/dL	0.3				▼	1.2	
Total Protein	7.17 g/dL	6.6	▼				8.3	

Figure 6-21. The patient continued to work out in the gym once daily but reduced the duration of the workout to 45 minutes. I gave him new nutritional instructions—to take protein supplements before and after training and before going to bed. Because the creatine kinase level was intensified, his muscles had been damaged due to lack of energy. He started treatment with T3 25 micrograms two times a day before he went to Dubai.

This was a classic example of the effect of carbs-rich meals before bed on nocturnal hormonal secretions and training in the gym after carbs instead of protein. It was written before!

Case 10: A 20-year-old woman with severe ADHD symptoms

During her childhood, this woman was beaten many times by her father because of her hyperactivity. She developed posttraumatic stress syndrome. Her parents were divorced. She had poor marks in school and was unable to finish high school because of reading problems. She cannot work because of depression , insomnia, and weakness. Her period is regular, but it is accompanied by heavy blood clots on the first day. She decided to study art and decorating to be able to find a job. Her lab studies report appears in Figure 6-22.

139

11.5 ··············· 22.7	12.3 pmol/l	**Free Thyroxine (FT4)**
3.5 ···········*······ 6.5	4.4 pmol/L	**Triiodothyronine Free FT3**
		הערות לבדיקה: החל מתאריך 18.9.22 חל
		שינוי
		בערכת הבדיקה.
		שים לב לעדכון ערכי.
		הייחוס
145 ··············· 619	686 nmol/l	**Cortisol 8 am (B)**
0.5 ···········*····· 4.8	2.93 mIu/l	**TSH**
		הערות לבדיקה: החל מתאריך 18.9.22 חל
		שינוי
		בערכת הבדיקה.
		שים לב לעדכון ערכי.
		הייחוס
0 ··········*······ 60	29 IU/ml	**Thyroid Peroxidase Ab**

Figure 6-22. Test results show that this 20-year-old woman with ADHD has a low FT4 level because her thyroid is "sick"; the FT3 is low because of problems with the T4/T3 conversion process due to the patient's stress level (her cortisol level is very high) The TSH (over 2) and the thyroid peroxidase Abs were high.

She probably has been suffering from Hashimoto hypothyroidism for a long time. She started treatment with T3 50 micrograms daily, a Paleo diet, and multivitamins and minerals, as well as melatonin and gamma-amino butyric acid 750 milligrams before sleep. She was also asked to monitor her body temperature and return for follow up. After 3 months of treatment, the patient's condition improved and her temperature rose to 36.8 at mid-day. The lab test showed the following results.

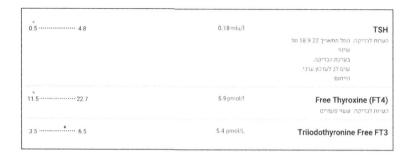

0.5 ··············· 4.8	0.18 mIu/l	**TSH** הערות לגדיקה: החל תחאריך 18.9.22 חל שינוי בערכת הבדיקה. שים לב לעדכון ערכי הייחוס
11.5 ··············· 22.7	5.9 pmol/l	**Free Thyroxine (FT4)** הערות לבדיקה: עשוי פעמיים
3.5 ·············· 6.5	5.4 pmol/L	**Triiodothyronine Free FT3**

Figure 6.23. shows an increased level of T3 to near its high level, the TSH is normal. But the T4 is low because the thyroid inflammation. She received several emotional treatments to promote relaxation using the NAET emotional approach.

141

Chapter 7

Thyroid Gland and Autoimmune Diseases

This chapter covers the cause of the development of autoimmune diseases in the body. As we have described many times throughout this book, the tiny thyroid gland has three main functions:

1. To keep the body temperature around 37 degrees Celsius (98.6 degrees Fahrenheit) so that proteins (including enzymes) can maintain their distinct three-dimensional shapes within body cells.
2. To produce energy particles (ATP; see Chapter 1).
3. To maintain the activity of the immune system.

Any slight change in the form of proteins in body tissues can disrupt the tissue's function. When the body is in a low-energy state, it directs ATPs in the immune system to provide the energy it needs to produce antibodies at the expense of other tissue functions. Fatigue and a low body temperature are the principal patient complaints after the acute period of the disease is over or with an autoimmune disease. A small change in body temperature (from 37 degrees to 36.5 degrees) is enough to slow down enzymatic activity in a specific area of the body.

The immune system is designed to deal with the invasion of bacteria, viruses, fungi, unidentified violent parasites that originate inside or outside the body, and substances released as a result of food sensitivities. It also has to deal with cancer cells that are produced daily in our bodies. The immune system consists of the thymus gland (located behind the sternum), the spleen (located behind the lower left section of the rib cage), lymph nodes (scattered throughout the body), and white blood cells. The thymus gland is designed to train white blood cells—called lymphocytes and monocytes—to identify and destroy any bacteria or viruses that enter the body or cancer cells that develop in the body. After undergoing this training, lymphocytes and monocytes are called natural killer—or NK—cells. Special tests are administered to identify their activity in the immune system. The thymus gland function depends on the levels of various hormones in the blood, particularly triiodothyronine (T3), insulin-like growth factor-1 (IGF-1), and the sex hormones. By the time we reach our 40s, the thymus gland has begun to shrink because of a decline in these hormones. At this point, the lymphocytes and monocytes start to lose their fighting ability. Therefore, when a person reaches menopause or andropause (that is, when the person enters the "third age"), there is an increased incidence of infectious diseases and cancer.

These invaders (bacteria, viruses, fungi, etc.) produce chemical substances that stimulate the activity of genes in the nucleus of the cell to produce proteins called cytokines. Cytokines are chemical messengers with a unique structure that reach the immune system to inform it of the presence of a foreign substance in the body. These unique proteins allow the immune system to identify the invader accurately so that they can produce specific antibodies to attack the specific invader. For example, the flu virus in winter causes the immune system to "wake up" and develop antibodies that can neutralize that virus. That's why we still feel good for a few days after the viral infection begins. There are two steps in the response of the immune system: (1) make a precise identification of the intruder; and (2) raise a specific response against the invader to weaken and eliminate its effect.

For example, in response to an intestinal condition, the thyroid gland's T3 hormone (its active hormone) triggers the secretion of immunoglobulin A (Ig A) in the intestines, where it binds to bacteria in the intestinal cavity to prevent them from penetrating the intestinal mucosa and entering the bloodstream.

During your lifetime, many invaders will enter your body; many of them will invade the body many times. During the first invasion, the immune system will neutralize them immediately. When an intruder enters the body a second time, the immune system will "remember" it and rapidly neutralize it. Sometimes the immune system prevents these invaders from spreading; as a result, they stay inside us for a long time (parasites, for example). This is how the system works against pests of foreign origin.

Under special conditions, the immune system can develop antibodies against the body's own cells and, thus, attack certain components of your body. This is how autoimmune diseases develop. All it takes is a tiny atomic change in the normal tissue structure in the body. The immune system recognizes the changed structure as alien and produces antibodies that are designed to attack it. When the immune system attacks a tissue in the body, signs of a local inflammatory process develop, including local fever, redness, swelling, pain, and structural changes in the tissue resulting in joint pain, rash, and other complaints specific to each disease. These diseases develop during the first 40 years of your life, a time when the immune system is very active. In the medical literature, only the symptoms and the effect of the immune system's attack on the body's tissues are described. I searched the literature to understand what causes the immune system to attack the affected tissue and possibly cause an autoimmune disease. The problem depends on the fact that although a lot of specific immune lab tests are performed, the clinician may forget that the hormonal system has some relationship with the disease. In this situation, when no connection is made between the autoimmune disease and the hormonal system, treatment is based on symptoms alone. If an incorrect treatment—for example, with steroids (prednisone, for example)—to relieved the pain and the local inflammation is started, the patient will continue to suffer for years.

I have listed here some of the many factors that can play a role in an autoimmune attack.

1. **Vitamins A and D:** We all know that vitamin D is related to bone metabolism. In recent years, however, studies have shown that there are receptors for vitamin D and for vitamin A on many cells in the immune system. It has been hypothesized that vitamins A and D are involved in many immunological processes, primarily in the prevention of autoimmune diseases. The importance of vitamins A and D increases a lot when we notice the link between a chronic deficiency in these vitamins in the general population and a high presence of many autoimmune diseases.

2. **Stress:** Many authors have considered the possibility that one of the reasons for the development of autoimmune diseases is a very high level of cortisol after the patient experiences a prolonged period of stress before getting sick. High levels of cortisol lower the T4/T3 conversion rate and disrupt the response of the immune system; this is suggested by the fact that many patients with an autoimmune disease

have low levels of T3 hormones and a high level of cortisol in the blood.

3. **Industrial oils** (polyunsaturated fatty acids, or PUFAs for short) contain many double bonds between carbon atoms (represented as C=C bonds) instead of the single bonds (C-C bonds) seen in saturated cholesterol fats. About 90% of the population uses these oils, which used to be defined by "experts" as healthy because they are extracted from sunflower, cotton, corn, grape and other seeds to produce canola and other liquid's oils. What are polyunsaturated fatty acids? They are found in fats that are extracted from agricultural grains. They are found in every food at a concentration of about 0.5 g per 100 milliliters (or cubic centimeters). Some are defined as trans or "healthy" trans fats. Many years ago, several studies claimed that saturated fats, such as the fat in butter—which does not have any double bonds—are unhealthy because they increase the risk of getting heart disease. Now it turned out that the liver produces cholesterol and saturated fats are extremely beneficial for general health, because the body used them to create the normally permeable membranes that surround the cell, the nucleus, and the mitochondrion. These membranes are composed of two layers of atomic molecules of cholesterol. The rise in blood cholesterol or glucose is caused by a decreased use of cholesterol by the mitochondria after a decrease in the production of T3, IGF-1, and sex hormones (which are created from cholesterol). In addition, PUFAs cause an increase in the production of free radicals that bond with low-density lipoprotein (LDL) cholesterol molecules and turns them into toxic substances. When the cells that form the inner lining (endothelium) of the arteries use PUFAs or oxidized LDL cholesterol to create energy, the resulting toxicity damages the endothelial

arterial walls, which, in turn, results in cholesterol plaque and gradual arterial blockage. These conditions usually occur after the age of 40, when the mitochondria and the glands themselves do not use cholesterol or glucose to create energy or the level of sex hormones produced is low. What is not often talked about is the most harmful effect of PUFAs in the body: the production of sealed membranes in or around the cell. These block the free entry of hormones and other substances into the cell and create resistance to the entry of T3 entry into the cell. In several studies in the medical literature, researchers reported that PUFAs cause additional damage during the production and use of thyroid hormones, specifically damage that reduces the T4/T3 conversion rate and blocks the entry of thyroid hormones into the cell, nucleus, and mitochondria. Thus, an entire population is always in a state of hypothyroidism and obesity (Figure 7-3).

The only monounsaturated fats (i.e., fats containing only one double [C=C] bond) that the body uses are olive oil coconut oil (in which most of the carbon bonds are saturated [C-C bonds]), and avocado oil (most [89%] of which is monounsaturated). As mentioned before, the fats in animals are mainly saturated fats. To maintain a normal lipid profile in the blood, a hormonal balance is necessary (see example in Chapter 8).

1. **Decrease in natural antioxidants:** For example, a lack of selenium can paralyze the activity of glutathione's SOD and other enzymes or food antioxidants, such as those minerals found in chocolate, green vegetables (including artichokes), shrimp's and many others. That are important for the immediate neutralization of free radicals and the 5'D function. They pass an electron to the free radical to reduce

its electrical instability (Figure 7.4). There is many sources of free radicals.

How antioxidants reduce free radicals

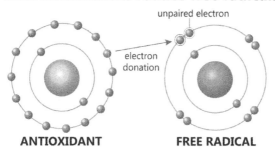

Figure 7.4. Interaction between free radicals and antioxidants. For details, please see Chapter 5).

When there are not enough antioxidants to neutralize the free radicals, the number of free radicals in the blood could increase dramatically. They can bond with any tissue in the body and change its structure, thereby triggering an immediate reaction by the immune system. Conventional medicine and HMOs pay little attention to the role of free radicals and the task of detecting them because of a lack of lab tests designed for that purpose (for example, for glycation.

2. **Glycation:** The attachment of a molecule of glucose to a protein is a natural phenomenon in the body. For example, glucose can bind with hemoglobin, a protein that is found in red blood cells. This particular connection is intensified in people who eat large amounts of carbohydrates and in patients with diabetes, in whom the glucose level in blood tends to rise. A blood test called the hemoglobin A1C (HbA1C)

test is used to measure the percentage of hemoglobin that is bound to glucose. The binding of glucose to hemoglobin (the glycation of hemoglobin) damages the normal structure of hemoglobin; as a result, it carries less oxygen to body tissues. The same process can occur in other body tissues, including the nervous system (for example, the retina) and the kidneys, where high levels of free radicals form as result of glycation and become the cause of complications of disease and the appearance of new symptoms. This vulnerability in some areas of the body is recognized by the immune system, which may attack and cause the appearance of an autoimmune disease.

3. **Leaky gut syndrome:** This condition is covered in our discussion of Hashimoto's disease (see Chapter 5). Patients with hypothyroidism often have many complaints related to the digestive system, especially people with a complete deficiency of IgA globulin.

Relationship between hypothyroidism and autoimmune diseases

In my opinion, there is a close connection between hypothyroidism and other hormonal diseases, including type 1 diabetes, type 2 diabetes, hypothyroidism, and Addison's disease.

• **Type 1 diabetes.** This condition, which usually develops during childhood, is considered an autoimmune disease. The conventional treatment is to modulate blood sugar levels only, even though antibodies against the thyroid gland and other organs in the body are increased in individuals with this disease. During the first 10 years of the disease, signs of hypothyroidism have been detected in about 10% of children by clinicians using standard diagnostic criteria. Children showing signs of hypothyroidism develop insulin resistance or other complications.

I believe that with an early diagnosis of hypothyroidism, it is possible to increase the number of children diagnosed with hypothyroidism in this population and prevent the complications of diabetes as much as possible. If hypoactivity is noted, the patient should be treated with T4. The patient's body temperature should be monitored throughout treatment period, because T4 can still be converted to T3 in children and is necessary for their normal development. If the T3 level falls below the upper limit of the normal range, the child should also receive T3 therapy. This will help them respond better to insulin and have fewer complications of the disease.

• **Hashimoto's disease** (Hashimoto's thyroiditis). Doctors usually start treatment of these patients with only 50 micrograms of T4 then soon see their patients return because the low rate of conversion of T4 to T3 allows them to still experience symptoms of hypothyroidism. Thus, it is advisable to give T3 only.

Graves' disease. In patients with this disease, antibodies are created that are identical in effect to the natural TSH hormone. This can cause TPO enzymes to become hyperactive, which may result in a very low production of natural TSH and increase the level of T4 and T3 (see case report in Chapter 6). After surgery or treatment with radioactive iodine, it is advisable to give patients only T3.

• **Celiac disease.** Symptoms of this condition, which is seen more frequently in children than in adults, are caused by hypersensitivity of the intestinal mucosa to gluten, a protein found in wheat. A local inflammation develops, along with abdominal pain, diarrhea, and disorders in the absorption of food elements that results in a leaky gut syndrome. A search of the medical literature shows that there is an awareness of the link between celiac disease and underactivity of the inflammation-fighting function of the thyroid gland and other hormonal problems. To find the link between celiac disease and hypothyroidism, it is advisable to measure TSH, FT3, and FT4 levels, as well as the levels of hormones secreted by other glands.

• **Type 2 diabetes.** Many adults with adult diabetes develop hypothyroidism and other hormone deficiencies. These may remain undiagnosed for some time because the only thyroid hormone that is measured is TSH. Additionally, diabetes interferes with the secretion of hormones at night; as a result, many patients with this disease have low levels of IGF-1, DHEA, and the sex hormones. Treatment with T3 and T4, together with hormonal balancing, will reduce resistance to insulin and most of the complications of this disease. The number of patients diagnosed with diabetes during adulthood or childhood will increase approximately 3.5 times in the next decade, because medical institutions do not currently address the causes of the disease and automatically push drugs—even those requiring special permission, as is needed for T3 test.

• **Addison's disease.** This rare disease is caused by an attack by the immune system on the adrenal glands—a pair of small glands that rest on top of the kidneys and secrete hormones that regulate salt, sugar, and sex hormone levels in the blood, as well as cortisol. Adrenal activity regulates blood pressure and stress. Interference with this activity in patients with Addison's disease is characterized by severe fatigue, weight loss, and darkening of skin color. According to Harrison's Textbook of Internal Medicine, common connections have been found between Addison's disease and hypothyroidism. The diagnosis is based on the results of laboratory measurements of adrenal hormones and other hormones that are present at extremely low levels in the blood.

• **Pernicious anemia.** Red blood cells are created in the bone marrow. The "parent cells" of the red blood cells need a lot of energy in the bone marrow to create hemoglobin; they also need vitamin B12. When antibodies attack the stomach lining, they interrupt the secretion of intrinsic factor, a protein that is necessary for vitamin B12 to be absorbed from the intestines. This results in pernicious anemia, which is characterized by a lack of red blood cells due to a lack of vitamin B12. In epidemiological studies, investigators have also found antibodies against the thyroid gland in this disease. It is not uncommon to discover antibodies against both diseases. Therefore, this type of anemia requires treatment for hypothyroidism as well as injections of vitamin B12.

• **Other autoimmune diseases.** Autoimmune diseases such as Raynaud's syndrome and Sjogren's syndrome usually appear as components of Hashimoto's disease. As autoimmune diseases, rheumatoid arthritis, lupus erythematosus, multiple sclerosis, scleroderma, and psoriasis have a connection with hypothyroidism. For example, I have found a high prevalence of hypothyroidism in patients with chronic fatigue syndrome, sarcoidosis, and fibromyalgia.

Treatment

Considering everything that has been said about the prevention or treatment of any autoimmune disease, we need to treat the digestive system first using digestive enzymes and probiotics then achieve a balance among hormonal secretions, if necessary, as well as provide the following supplements: collagen 100 grams per day, vitamin D 5000 International Units per day, vitamin A (eat two or more carrots a day), vitamin E (from avocados or a supplement of 400 International Units per day), and glutathione from NAC supplements of 1000 to 2000 milligrams per day, along with appropriate doses of probiotics, selenium, iron, magnesium, zinc, and the vitamin B complex. Patients may also benefit from a low dose (20-40 milligrams) of progesterone and T4, with or without T3 (according to body temperature), as well as an increase in deeply colored fruits and vegetables for antioxidants. In addition, these patients should reduce their consumption of simple carbohydrates to 100 to 150 grams per day, avoid PUFAS as much as possible, and reduce stress.

In conclusion: For any patient who is diagnosed with one or more of the autoimmune diseases described in this chapter, it is advisable to perform a comprehensive test of thyroid hormones and enzymes—including TSH, FT3, FT4, Anti-TPO Ag, and Anti-TG Ag—and decipher the test results according to the criteria I have established to increase the chance of an accurate diagnosis. Complementary treatment should be provided according to the criteria of functional medicine. You can use Table 4-1 to find the desired level of hormones at the age of 20. Complementary hormonal treatment will improve each patient's condition and reduce the severity of disease. It should also be noted that every patient who comes to a hospital with a serious illness develops hypothyroidism, because the illness will suppress the hypothalamus-pituitary-thyroid axis.

Case Presentation

S.P. is a 30-year-old woman complaining of dry skin, cold feet and hands, a slow pulse, an irregular menstrual cycle with heavy bleeding and pain, a fungal infection, infertility, severe fatigue, hair loss, various allergies, asthma attacks, muscle and joint pain, a body temperature of 36.0 to 36.5 degrees, and other nonspecific complaints.

TEST NAME	VALUE	UNITS	NORMAL RANGE
TPO Ag	165	IU/mL	0..............................35*
Iron	75	µg/dL	60...*......................126
Vitamin B12	318	pg/dL	211....*................911
TSH	1.19	mIU/dL	0.95..*.........................4.7
FT4	1.0	ng/dL	0.8......*.........................1.9
FT3	86.0	ng/dL	72...*......................170
DHEA	6.12	µmol/L	0.7......*.......................12.5
Vitamin D	17.9	µg/L	30.0*........................100
Estradiol	222	pmol/L	N/A
Progesterone	2.61	nmol/L	N/A
P/E2 ratio	12.6	less than 50	N/A

Figure 7-4. Abbreviations: DHEA, dehydroepiandrosterone; FT3, free triiodo-thyronine; FT4, free thyroxine; P/E2, progesterone/estradiol ratio; TPO, thyroid peroxidase; TSH, thyroid stimulating hormone.

Diagnosis: This patient has Hashimoto's disease. Her iron, vitamin D, and vitamin B12 levels are in the low to low-normal range due to severe menstrual bleeding and absorption disorders. Although her TSH is normal, her FT4 level is below the central range. Either her thyroid gland is not secreting enough T4 or not converting it to FT3 due to a problem with 5'D activity. Her progesterone/estradiol ratio (P/E2 ratio) is less than 50, and she has estradiol dominance syndrome (see Chapter 8).

Chapter 8

Disorders of the Woman's Menstrual Cycle

During a woman's lifetime, she learns to receive the menstrual period as a natural event that permits her to know if she is able to get pregnant or if she is not still within her fertile age. The menstrual cycle should last 2 to 3 days with the loss of a small amount of blood (estimated at 20-35 cc) and mild abdominal pain. According to Our Bodies, Ourselves: A New Edition for a New Era, this natural event starts to change slowly to a heavy period with severe abdominal pain and changes in the woman's attitude. Some look for relief; others prefer to stop the menstrual cycle temporarily by taking hormone pills. Later in life, at about age 40 to 50, the woman may find that she can't get pregnant because of physical changes that occurred without her knowing it. She begins to gain weight, feels mild bouts of depression, her sex drive is not what it used to be, she has trouble sleeping at night, she gets tired easily, and sometimes she suffers from headaches, profuse night sweats, and hair loss. Additionally, her menstrual cycle has completely changed—sometimes with minor and irregular bleeding. At some point in life, every woman knows that she goes through physical and mental changes that are the result of hormonal imbalances in her body, one of which causes her menstrual cycle to be different from her cycle during puberty. She accepts these changes as natural events, however, events that take place because she is a woman.

After she has finished raising her children, a woman tries to feel fulfilled by looking for new horizons. She may look for a new job or an occupation that interests her, and she must be healthy to fulfill her mission. New changes begin to appear, however—not short, strong, and dramatic changes, such as those that took place during puberty, but prolonged changes that include signs of severe mental and physical disorders that are accompanied by new and troublesome symptoms. It should be noted that these changes can appear at any point in a woman's life. For convenience, I have divided them into three periods:

• **First period:** Disturbances in the menstrual cycle may occur at a young age (17-30 years)—the age of fertility during which her monthly cycle is still in place. Severe symptoms then appear during menstruation or shortly before the development of premenstrual syndrome.

• **Second period:** This stage is marked by complaints that a woman expresses during her 30s and 40s, when she feels the changes in her body that foretell what is to come and the symptoms that appear just before her menstrual cycle. She has stopped taking pills, she is having difficulty getting pregnant, she may have had an abortion, or her menstrual cycle may have become irregular (the premenopausal period).

• **Third period:** From her 50s on, with partial or complete cessation of her menstrual cycle, a woman becomes aware of disturbing symptoms that will accompany her for a long time. These symptoms herald the coming of menopause

First stage: premenstrual syndrome

The symptoms of premenstrual syndrome appear before or during the menstrual cycle at the age of 15 to 30 years. During this period of life, the balance between the sex hormones estradiol and progesterone begins to change, even though there is still an orderly cycle and ovulation. In most cases, the woman accepts these phenomena as normal, without noticing that there has been any change from what was before. That's why I want to describe how changes in the cycle develop. If she understands what is happening during this period of time, she can alleviate these symptoms and understand why her body has changed. But first she has to learn about the hormones that manage a normal menstrual cycle to achieve appropriate hormone levels when something goes wrong when she takes non-natural hormones.

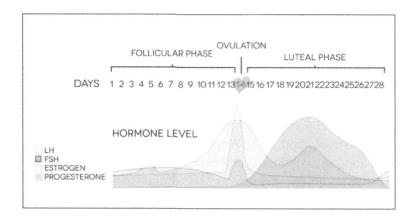

Figure 8-1. Diagram of the hormonal regulation of the menstrual cycle.

159

During the first 14 days after bleeding ends, estradiol levels increase (blue color) as a result of the effect of FSH (green color). During this period of time, the woman's eggs (ova) mature to contain 23 genes. On the 15th day of the cycle, ovulation occurs under the influence of LH yellow color) and FSH (green color). The egg (ovum) is now "ripe" and ready to meet with sperm cells. During the second half of the cycle, the progesterone level rises (red color), the libido gets stronger, and the body temperature rises, reaching 36.7 to 37.0 degrees Celsius, to let her know she is in the second part of the cycle. During this period of time, her progesterone level should be 50 times higher (red color) than her estradiol level (blue color) to prepare the inner lining of her uterus (endometrium) with nutrients and other materials needed by the fertilized egg. If the egg is not fertilized, the lining of the uterus is shed, bleeding starts, and the woman knows she is not pregnant. For a woman to conceive, her body temperature must be around 37 degrees, her uterus must be able to function like an incubator, the endometrium must be well developed, and her progesterone level must be 50 times higher than her estradiol level. Under these conditions, the uterus is ready to receive and grow the fertilized egg.

The most common menstruation-related complaints during the fertile period

During this period, there are complaints described as thyroid underactivity and a menstrual disorder collectively known as premenstrual syndrome (PMS), which is characterized by severe abdominal pain just before or during the period itself. The patient complains about heavy bleeding, which includes clotted blood, which, in turn, causes iron deficiency anemia; excessive irritability, fatigue, anxiety attacks, or depression; confused thoughts; headaches or migraines; dizziness, fainting, and the inability to concentrate; joint pain, back pain, and swelling in the legs and face; stomach bloating, gas, a craving for sweet food; cold hands and feet; hypersensitivity; and swollen breasts. The adult woman is unable to get pregnant or has had repeated miscarriages, recurrent urinary tract infections, asthma attacks, allergies, acne, sleep disorders, and the appearance of an auto-immune disease.

The main cause of premenstrual syndrome is a **hormonal imbalance due to excessive estradiol compared with progesterone during the second part of the period.** We live in a very toxic environment, with toxins in food, in the air, or in substances for personal use that can affect the hormonal system, especially the thyroid gland.

1. In the second part of the cycle, an imbalance between progesterone and estradiol occurs immediately after ovulation (Figure 8-1). There is also a high level of estradiol compared with progesterone; thus, the ratio between them changes. In other words, the endometrial mucosa does not have the conditions necessary to absorb the fertilized egg. During the second part of the cycle, the concentration of progesterone is normally 50 times higher than that of estradiol, but the ratio between progesterone and estrogen (the P/E2 ratio) is less than 50—and she can't be pregnant.

2. Another factor that can interfere with the menstrual cycle is hidden hypoactivity (low T3 syndrome). This may develop because the woman is under constant stress, eats high-carbohydrate foods, or uses cosmetics containing substances that disturb the T4/T3 conversion rate. As a result, the ovaries do not have enough energy to produce progesterone. The uterus only serves as an incubator; if the woman suffers from thyroid hypoactivity and the body temperature is lower than 36.7 degrees, the fetus cannot develop and the pregnancy may come to an end.

3. If the woman suffers from estradiol control (high levels of estradiol compared with progesterone) during the second part of her cycle, the cycle will be difficult and prolonged because of a very thickened mucosa that does not contain the nutrients needed by the fetus. Estradiol causes the mucous cells to divide many times and penetrate the uterine muscles. In advanced cases, these cells spread throughout the uterus. As a result, bleeding becomes profuse, with blood clots and severe contractions of the uterus, the latter occurring because the uterine muscle has developed excessively and the uterus needs to get rid of blood clots. If heavy bleeding occurs every month for an extended period of time, the thickening of the endometrium can lead to a disease called endometriosis and, in turn, to the formation of benign myomas within the uterine muscles or the development of cysts in the ovaries and breasts. When the situation is not as it should be, very disturbing physical phenomena occur. The woman may seek relief by taking pills to reduce the pain or by lying in bed until the symptoms pass. Her mood changes, family relationships go wrong, or she asks for help from a gynecologist. Some women prefer to take pills to stop the disturbing period completely.

4. This health condition usually leads to increased stress and, thus, an increase in the level of cortisol in the blood. Many women with this condition complain about symptoms resembling those of thyroid dysfunction, which are described in Chapter 4. The main effect of cortisol is on 5'D enzyme activity in the liver and kidneys. As a result, the level of T3 in the blood decreases, and the process of eliminating toxins in the liver goes wrong—especially the process of eliminating the hormone estradiol. The estradiol metabolite, when not removed from the body, might interfere with the function of the thyroid gland, causing Hashimoto's disease, Graves' dis-

ease, or another autoimmune disease.

5. Exposure to chemical substances that have an effect similar to that of estradiol (i.e., an estrogenic effect) can have the same results as exposure to phytoestrogens. These substances are derived from soybeans, flaxseeds, unsaturated sesame oil, and chickpeas, all of which contain varying amounts of phytoestrogens. Phytoestrogens have two effects on the body: (1) Because their chemical structure is similar to that of estradiol, they compete with natural estradiol for its receptors on the cell surface, thereby elevating the estradiol level in the blood; and (2) they bind with estrogen receptors, thereby reducing the symptoms but without having the same natural biological effect as estradiol. In both cases, estradiol levels in the blood remain high because the cells do not use it. High estradiol levels suppress thyroid activity.

6. Xenoestrogens (xenon is derived from the Greek, meaning "foreign") are substances found in the environment that are extracted from petroleum and other synthetic industrial substances such as the pesticide DDT (also known as dichlorodiphenyltrichloroethane); PBBs (polybrominated biphenyls), which are found in many plastic materials used in the home; BPA (bisphenol A) and PCBs (polychlorinated biphenyls), both of which are widely used in plastics; and PPD (paraphenylenediamine), a material used in hair dyes and cosmetics. The materials used in plastics are found in plastic boxes, cutlery, and bottles, as well as DVDs, CDs, toys, and printing paper. When hot water is used to clean plastic materials, their toxins can easily leak into any food and drink in those containers. Cosmetics and perfumes are often used daily. They have a powerful estrogenic effect and can even be toxic or allergenic. They can change the structure of body tissues and the standard structure of the DNA, resulting in genetic mutations and cancer. Compared with natural es-

tradiol, which has a short period of action and is neutralized in the liver, these substances bind to the estradiol receptor for a long time and cause the increased production of free radicals. In short: Be careful!

7. These changes can lead to mood changes, sharp fluctuations in blood sugar levels, and an addiction to carbohydrates. Women who undergo these changes need to eat soon after their blood sugar drops. Unconscious mental restlessness develops between meals, leading to increased cortisol secretion and a desire for carbohydrates.(see Figure 1-6)

8. Treatment with drugs or pills: Treatment with drugs that contain unnatural hormones to regulate the cycle, prevent pregnancy, ameliorate depression and other mental disorders, or prevent heartburn can worsen the hormonal imbalance, leading to the visible development of hypothyroidism. After these drugs raise the cortisol level, they paralyze 5'D activity and elevate the level of free radicals. As a result, T3 levels decrease and the body temperature drops to less than 36.5 degrees during the second part of the cycle (Figures 8-2 , 8-3 and 8-4).

9. Development of inflammatory processes: During this period of life, a woman may develop various inflammatory processes or autoimmune diseases. Inflammatory processes increase free radical, cortisol, and estradiol levels in the blood and reduce progesterone and T3 levels. One of the important things that contribute a lot to the development of inflammatory processes is the use of drugs that contain unnatural hormones to treat or prevent pregnancy, as well as unsaturated oils, industrial fats (for example, canola oil), trans fats, or deep-fried foods. Such factors lead to a deficiency in zinc, magnesium, vitamins A and C, and the B vitamins, all of which are necessary to create thyroid hormones and support mitochondrial function.

10. Excess weight: Addiction to carbohydrates and weight gain increase the activity of the enzyme aromatase in fat cells, increasing estradiol and insulin levels in the blood by 30%.

Test Name	Results	Units	Reference Value	Normal Range
Cortisol	573	nmol/L	138-690	..........,,*.
DHEA-s	8.06	mmol/L	0.95-11.7	.......*....
Estradiol	452	mpmol/L	250-786	.......*....
FSH	11.8	mIU/L	1.5-9.	............*
LH	16.4	miU/L	0.5-56.90	.....*......
Progesterone	4.8	nmol/mL	8-58	*...........
IGF-1	359	nmol/L	163-584	.....*......

Figure 8-2. Results of blood tests for a 17-year-old adolescent with complaints consistent with premenstrual syndrome. The results of these tests, which were performed on the 21st day of her menstrual cycle, show a high level of estradiol (452 picomol/L) compared with progesterone (4.8 nanomol/L). The P/E2 ratio is 10.6 (4.8 ÷ 0.452). She is stressed because of personal problems and eats a lot of carbohydrates (which she has done so for many years). This results in a cortisol level that is in the upper limit of the normal range instead of the lower half. FSH and LH are high because the pituitary gland "pushes" the ovaries to secrete more estradiol and progesterone. Abbreviations: DHEA, dehydroepiandrosterone; FSH. follicle-stimulating hormone; LH, luteinizing hormone.

165

Test Name	Results	Units	Reference Value	Normal Range
Estradiol	Les than 70	pmol/L	259-786	*..............
TSH	4	PmmIU.L	0.55-4.78	...........*....
FT4	13.6	pmol/L	10-20	......*........
Prolactin	170.1	mgram/mL	less of 25	..............*
Progesterone	Less than 1.7	nmol/L	8.58	*..............
Cortisol	832	nmol/L	138-690	..............*

Figure 8-3. Results of tests given to the patient discussed in Figure 8-2 after treatment with progesterone and DHEA. She felt calm and exhibited an increase in both of these hormones and symptom relief. Also, her P/E2 ratio now exceeds 50 (40.4 ÷ 0.479=84.42). Abbreviations: DHEA, dehydroepiandrosterone; FSH, follicle-stimulating hormone; LH, luteinizing hormone.

At this stage of premenstrual syndrome, a woman's symptoms can be severe enough to disrupt her studies and her marriage and other interpersonal relationships. The following changes occur in the brain: High Estradiol produces less GABA (short for gamma amino butyric acid) and more serotonin. Both of these are electrical conductors in the brain: GABA reduces and suppresses pain; high serotonin levels can lead to mental restlessness. That is why these patients experience outbreaks of mental restlessness, along with sleep problems. Due to an increase in estradiol, blood vessels expand and migraine attacks, dizziness, low blood pressure, or chest pain can appear.

The conventional treatment in these cases is based on symptoms only. Medication to regulate the cycle causes a decrease in the production of sex hormones in the ovaries (Figure 8-4). Because the menstrual cycle is now under the control of synthetic hormones, many side effects appear and the cortisol level rises. Again, these treatments lead to a decrease in T3 levels because they affect 5'D activity.

Test Name	Results	Units	Reference Value	Normal Range
Estradiol	Les than 70	pmol/L	259-786	*..............
TSH	4	PmmIU.L	0.55-4.78	.............*....
FT4	13.6	pmol/L	10-20	......*........
Prolactin	170.1	mgram/mL	less of 25	.............*
Progesterone	Less than 1.7	nmol/L	8.58	*..............
Cortisol	832	nmol/L	138-690	.............*

Figure 8-4. A 30-year-old woman taking birth control pills is being treated with 50 micrograms eltroxin to relieve symptoms of hypothyroidism. The laboratory test results show very low levels of estradiol and progesterone, indicating ovarian inactivity due to the use of birth control pills. We also see an increase in cortisol and prolactin, indicating stress. Her TSH level is higher than 1.5, which indicates thyroid underactivity, and her T4 level is below the middle level, despite treatment. It is possible that T4 was not absorbed well because of local problems in the intestines. The T3 hormone was not tested. The level of synthetic hormones cannot be measured using standard laboratory tests. Abbreviations: FT4, free thyroxine; T3, triiodothyronine; TSH, thyroid stimulating hormone.

Treatments for various psychological conditions—such as stress, depression, or epilepsy—or even after dental procedures can cause thyroid hypoactivity. Years after these pills have been used, breast cancer might appear.

Because natural hormones are destroyed in the stomach or during the digestive process, drug companies, through chemical manipulation, changed the structure of progesterone so that it can be taken orally (Utrogestan). But the liver has to release progesterone from this chemical so that it can get into the bloodstream. This process places a heavy load on the liver and can cause an increase in liver enzymes on blood tests. In the end, the patient may be forced to stop taking these drugs and continue to experience menstrual disorders. Utrogestan can be replaced with other medications. It is wise to use progesterone cream 40 to 80 milligrams daily; this product may be purchased on the internet.

After we know the cause of this phenomenon, we only need to restore the ratio of progesterone to estradiol to its normal level (as determined by nature) during the next menstrual period; this can be done by changing our lifestyle and diet. For this reason, it is advisable to measure estrogen and progesterone levels on day 18 to 24 of the cycle (see Figure 8-1). The progesterone level should be lower than the estrogen level so that the P/E2 ratio (progesterone/estradiol ratio) is less than 50 (sometimes 5-20) (Figures 8-2 and 8-3) after progesterone treatment. Next, the patient's body temperature should be checked orally or using a digital thermometer (see Chapter 3), and the necessary laboratory tests should be performed. Ask your doctor to perform lab tests for the following items: TSH, FT3, FT4, Anti-TPO Ag, Anti-TG Ag, estradiol, progesterone; cortisol 8 am, LH, FSH, prolactin, and DHEA, as well as general blood studies for glucose and cholesterol, as well as a complete blood cell panel.

Suppose the test results show a high estradiol level compared with progesterone that results in a P/E2 ratio of less than 50. In that case, you should be given hormone replacement therapy in the form of a natural progesterone ointment cream (not pills) that can be applied all over your body immediately after ovulation—from day 15 day of your cycle until day 26 or day 27. The dosage is 20 milligrams in the morning and another 20 milligrams in the evening. This treatment will increase the level of progesterone compared with estradiol. During the second part of the cycle in the following month and while she is being treated with progesterone, the woman should undergo another estradiol-progesterone lab study on appropriate days (day 18-day 24) to check the progesterone level and evaluate her condition (Figure 8-3). The progesterone cream should be applied after the blood sample has been taken.

If the blood test that is taken during the second month shows that the P/E ratio has not reached 50, the progesterone dose must be increased to 40 milligrams twice a day during the next cycle until the menstrual cycle feels comfortable. Thus, we search for the appropriate dose of biological hormones until the menstrual cycle returns to normal (Figure 8-3). In addition to treating the biological hormone imbalance, it is necessary to treat the factors that led to this phenomenon; that is, to change eating habits, reducing the intake of carbohydrates to a total of 100 to 150 grams per day consumed during morning and afternoon hours only. A small protein dinner is recommended before sleep mainly to increase the amount of tyrosine (an amino acid found in chicken that serves as a raw material for making thyroid hormones). She should exercise after mid-day during 45 minutes; take 50 grams of protein powder to increase the IGF-1 level and reduce the cortisol level, and then have a good sleep the next night. It is also advisable to avoid fried foods as much as possible, especially at dinner, and to reduce stress, take a multivitamin along with zinc, selenium and magnesium supplements, and create a diet based on natural foods by avoiding industrial oils (such as canola oil), eating fresh vegetables and fruits, and using olive oil. This protocol may not be easy, but it prevents disease for those who love themselves and want to reach the third age with maximum vitality.

It should be noted that this hormonal treatment is temporary and can only be provided for about 6 months if the woman changes her lifestyle. Her menstrual cycle will return to its regular course, with mild pain and light bleeding for 3 to 4 days. If the cycle returns to the same as it was before the treatment, the woman should follow the treatment for a longer period of time, with more emphasis on changing her lifestyle.

This is the time when a woman wants to get pregnant. Because of the hormonal imbalance I described, however, she may not have been successful in this. The instructions I mentioned can be used to balance the temperature and condition of the endometrium. After treatment for the estradiol dominance syndrome and thyroid underactivity, she can become pregnant.

The perimenopausal period

When a woman reaches her forties, she may find herself in a state of chronic stress because of the pressure placed on her by society and work to be efficient in her home and in her professional life. Some women choose an extreme or vegetarian diet to lose weight, some smoke, some decide to get pregnant after they stop taking birth control pills, or even after chemotherapy or other types of treatment. Often the signs of premenopausal represent a continuation of menstrual disorders that began during her fertile age or simply herald the arrival of menopause.

During this period of prolonged stress, the cortisol level rises to the upper third of the normal range and sometimes beyond it instead of remaining in the lower third. The result is an increase in estradiol. The progesterone and DHEA levels are within the lower limit of the normal range, as are the thyroid hormones. Because the woman gained weight, her aromatase (also known as estrogen synthetase) enzymes are producing more estradiol. In any case, if we calculate the P/E2 ratio again, the result will be less than 50.

Because of a high level of cortisol and an increased appetite, the woman gains weight and her blood test results show a high level of glucose and/or cholesterol in the blood. She also craves sweets; and when her blood sugar level drops, she complains of memory loss, fatigue, and muscle weakness. She also experiences fluid and salt retention, which leads to an increase in blood pressure and a decrease in progesterone, along with adverse conditions associated with a relatively high level of estrogen compared with progesterone from the age of 40 years to 65 years. This phenomenon affects her mentally and physically.

To find relief from her symptoms, she goes to various doctors and takes many tests. She is sometimes told that the laboratory test results are normal for a woman her age and that everything she complains about is "in her head." The complaints I described in the previous section continue in this patient, and she is now given tranquilizers, drugs with unnatural synthetic hormones, and antidepressants. After many years of high doses of estradiol, a gynecological examination reveals precancerous changes in the cervix or a benign fibroid tumor (myoma) that causes heavy monthly bleeding. It is then recommended that the uterus should be removed. In other tests, cysts are found in her ovaries or breasts.

The effect of drugs containing hormones to prevent pregnancy: Usually a drug that is introduced to prevent pregnancy is based on a new molecule that was invented by a drug company and is not found in the human body. For its efforts, the company may receive rewards. When a woman receives treatment with such artificial hormones, her symptoms are relieved, despite the fact that the medication has no biological effect. She is not receiving treatment with natural biological hormones, however. The prolonged effect of pills with synthetic hormones may only result in the development of inflammatory factors (for example, through an increase in free radicals), as well as the appearance of genital cancer or endometriosis (the spread of endometrial tissue to the abdomen) or osteoporosis or osteopenia.

All of the conditions I have described are related to the effect of many years of excess estradiol that is not restrained by progesterone during the second part of the cycle, as well as hidden underactivity of the thyroid gland or prolonged treatment with birth control pills. In my opinion, everything looks fine if the woman controls her period, but the body does not respond well after a long period of using pills. Various symptoms will appear, and sometimes pills are expensive—not only in terms of money, but also in terms of the risk for blood clots, cancer, endometriosis, and weight gain.

Measuring the body temperature in the morning and afternoon to determine the thyroid gland's activity can clarify why a woman does not get pregnant or why she has a miscarriage (as described in Chapter 3). Because of all the hormonal changes and changes in dietary habits during this period, a woman may gain weight, mainly in the hips, buttocks, calves, and stomach.

During these years, women often complain about the symptoms we described earlier, including water retention (edema) and weight gain, because of the increased production of estradiol in fat cells (Figure 8-6).

To prove my point, I found surveys in the literature that were designed to determine whether birth control pills, which contain synthetic non-natural hormones, increase the incidence of cancer. Giersch and colleagues (2013) reviewed the medical literature on this subject from 2000 to 2013. The incidence of breast, cervical, endometrial, and colon cancer was investigated. They found a significantly increased risk for cancer in women who received these drugs compared with women who did not take them. Women who used to have free sex while taking birth control pills became infected with the papilloma virus in the cervix. It should be noted that the effect of the pill over very long periods was not tested.

This is the place to point out that hormone replacement therapy using biological hormones that are 100% identical to those in humans (these are called bio-identical) is beneficial for the body when given after laboratory monitoring. They do not cause cancer, and when there is a hormonal balance, cancer can be prevented, because, together with T3, they strengthen the immune system. Practitioners of conventional medicine usually do not check for this possibility on days 18 to 24 of the cycle. As we saw before, the lack of biological hormone treatment leads to the development of diabetes, high cholesterol, weight gain, cardiovascular diseases, and other diseases because the glands that produce sex hormones stop using cholesterol as a raw material.

The findings of "estradiol hormone dominance syndrome" in this group

A woman diagnosed with estradiol dominance syndrome has the following health risks: precancerous changes in the uterine cervix or endometrium, myoma in the uterus, ovarian and breast cysts, uterine or breast cancer, allergies of various types, endometriosis, an autoimmune disease such as lupus (systemic lupus erythematosus, or SLE), inflammation of the thyroid gland (Hashimoto's syndrome), hypothyroidism, obesity, an increase in cortisol and decrease in DHEA, and subsequent diseases. What are the signs and symptoms of prolonged estradiol dominance syndrome? Women with this syndrome complain about abnormal menstrual cycles marked by heavy and painful periods—a sign of PMS (Figure 8-7).

Name	Results	Units	Reference Range	Average Range
ESTRADIOL	131	pmol/L	less 100	.........*
LH	35.8	IU/L	0.56-14	..........*
FSH	46.3	IU/L	0-0.6	.... *
PROGESTERONE	less1.7	ng/mL	5-20	*...........
TESTOSTERONE TOTAL	less0.9	pmol/L	8.4-28.7	*..........
AGF-1	10.4	nmol/L	3.51-28.99	..*..........
DHEA-S	0.77	mmol.L	0.9-11.6	*...........
CORTISOL	564	nmol/L	038-690	.........*....

Figure 8-7. This is the hormone lab report for a 45-year-old woman with gallstones who presented with complaints of symptoms of premenopause and a regular period. Blood tests were performed on the 20th day of her period. The test shows estradiol dominance syndrome, with a low progesterone level (less than 1.7 nanomoles per liter compared with 131 picomoles per liter of estradiol). That means her P/E2 ratio was 12.97 (1.7 ÷ 0.131) instead of 50 or more. You can also see a significant decrease in DHEA and increase in LH and FSH. Estradiol is produced when the enzyme aromatase acts on cholesterol in fat cells to convert it to estradiol. The cortisol level is high because the woman is under covert stress; the DHEA and progesterone levels are low because they are being converted to cortisol. Abbreviations: DHEA, dehydroepiandrosterone; FSH, follicle-stimulating hormone; IGF-1, insulin-like growth hormone-1; LH, luteinizing hormone.

Because of the risk for weight gain, women with menstrual disorders should avoid conventional treatment with nonbiological hormones or an intrauterine device with hormones and should avoid taking antidepressants or other drugs.

Another problem with a high estradiol level is that the estradiol level in the blood does not reflect the estradiol level in the cell. Researchers found that the concentration of estradiol in the uterine lining is 50 times higher in the uterine cells than in the blood. This situation may exist in many tissues of the body. This finding is significant, because if the enzymes responsible for neutralizing the toxic effects of estradiol cannot offset estradiol levels because of a lack of energy to remove it from the body, estradiol metabolite levels will rise in every tissue over a long period of time. This can damage the DNA, causing mutations and triggering the initiation of cancer. High levels of estradiol metabolites have been found in various types of cancer. After women received resveratrol and an NAC supplement, the level of toxic estradiol metabolites was significantly reduced. The following questions remain, however: (1) Is this a mechanism that causes cancer in the body; and (2) is it possible to reduce the incidence of cancer by using these supplements?

Tests related to the premenopausal state

Once we understand that all of the symptoms of menopause are related to an imbalance between progesterone and estradiol, we need to perform the following laboratory tests: TSH, FT3, FT4, DHEA-S, total testosterone, estradiol, progesterone, insulin, HbA1C, CR, prolactin, cortisol 8 am, anti-TPO Ag, and Anti TG Ag. These blood tests should be performed at some point between day 18 and day 24 of her menstrual cycle, because this is when the progesterone level is expected to be the highest compared to estradiol (Figures 8-1 and 8-7).

The treatment is similar to the one described earlier: Start by applying progesterone cream at a dose of 20 milligrams twice a day from day 15 of the cycle until day 26. If your symptoms do not improve in the current cycle, repeat the treatment during the next cycle, increasing the progesterone dose to 40 milligrams twice a day starting on day 15. To tell if your condition is improving, have blood tests for estradiol and progesterone performed at some point between days 18 and 24 of the cycle. The P/E2 ratio should be greater than 50; otherwise, the dose should be adjusted as needed. Usually if the symptoms have improved, this treatment can be continued for life.

Menopause

When a woman is around the age of 45 years, the picture of menopause becomes more turbulent. This is a common phenomenon in industrialized countries but not in Asian agricultural regions, where the environment is calm, the air is clean, exposure to xenoestrogens is low, the typical diet is based on plant foods containing phytoestrogens, and most of the residents are involved in agricultural work. This lifestyle helps minimize symptoms of menopause and mitigates the phenomenon of premenopausal or menopause itself. By contrast, menopause is considered the end of a woman's sexual life in Western urban areas. As a result, various personal problems may arise. Additionally, woman living in Western urban areas are exposed to environmental toxins that have "estradiol-like" effects; unhealthy foods rich in sugar; an unhealthy lifestyle; and synthetic hormones in cosmetics, and drugs, as well as synthetic agents used to prevent weight gain and other preventable problems. The main complaints during this period are hot flashes and profuse sweating, especially at night; weight gain, which does not decrease despite various diets; urinary incontinence and recurrent infections in the urinary tract or vagina; change in mood; lack of sleep; low sex drive; palpitations; pain during intercourse due to vaginal dryness; clouding of thoughts; excessive irritability, depression or panic attacks; fatigue, shortness of breath with light exertion; sadness and crying for no apparent reason; bone pain due to calcium loss; osteopenia or osteoporosis; chest pain; headache and migraine; decreased memory and inability to concentrate; varicose veins in the legs; pain in the joints, especially in the knees and shoulders; and hair loss. All of these phenomena develop gradually.

Some women with these complaints turn to doctors for help because they suspect they have developed some disease. They are sent for a series of tests to find any new diseases and to receive conventional drug treatment. All of these complaints, however, are related to three things: (1) continued imbalance among various hormones; (2) a permanent decrease in important sex hormones; and (3) hidden or overt hypoactivity of the thyroid and other endocrine glands.

Signs of hormonal deficiency

Progesterone levels decrease more rapidly than estradiol levels between the ages of 40 and 50 years (Figure 8-5). During menopause, the ovaries stop secreting these two hormones. Thyroid hormone levels remain low beginning at this time of life. As a result, the skin looks thin and wrinkled. Many wrinkles appear on the face, especially around the mouth; breasts droop and shrink; joint and bone problems develop, along with high blood pressure; vaginal dryness develops, causing difficulty during sex; nails become brittle; cholesterol and triglyceride levels increase; back bends become very difficult because of osteoporosis or osteopenia; overt diabetes appears, along with weight gain; and the body temperature falls below 37 degrees Celsius.

Based on all of these conditions, the patient is "diagnosed" with the presence of menopause (Figure 8-8).

NAME OF TEST	RESULTS	AVERAGE RANGE
Cortisol	353 nmol/L	118(......*.......)618
DHEA	1.88 mmol/L	0.95(..*............)11.7
FT4	12.2 pmol/L	10.3(..*...........)19.7
FT3	4.32 pmol/L	3.5(.....*.........)6.5
TSH	10.74 mIU/L	0.5(................)*4.8
Estradiol	<100 pmol/L	250(...............)786
Progesterone	<2 nmol/L	1.5(................)9.1
FSH	93.2	LESS THAN 3 IU
LH	41.4	[in the lower third] LESS THAN 3 IU
Insulin	15	[in the lower third] LESS THAN 10 IU

Figure 8-8. Results of a hormonal study of a 52-year-old woman who has not had a menstrual period for 3 years and exhibits symptoms of menopause. These results show a lack of estrogen and progesterone, low levels of DHEA and T3, an increase in TSH (an expression of hypothyroidism, which often accompanies menopause), and an insulin level just over 10 mIU/L (milli-international units per liter), which indicates latent diabetes. Abbreviations: DHEA, dehydroepiandrosterone; FT3, free triiodothyronine; FT4, free thyroxine; FSH, follicle-stimulating hormone; LH, luteinizing hormone; TSH, thyroid-stimulating hormone.

So what are you to do?

Before starting hormone replacement therapy, a menopausal woman will need laboratory blood tests like the ones we requested for premenopausal women, as well as general tests. A gynecological examination and ultrasound of the abdomen and the carotid neck arteries is also required to rule out any arteriosclerotic disease or a cancerous process. Because a menopausal woman does not have a monthly period, the blood test can be performed at any time, all year round. The test results can be compared with the placement of the asterisk in Table 4-1 or Figure 8-8. Usually, hormone levels correspond with those seen between the age of 50 to 60 years. We need to raise them to levels seen in the middle column. Biotechnology companies will produce progesterone, estradiol, and any other hormone that the body needs, including T3, T4, and DHEA. These are available as a cream, gel, or tablet, depending on the hormone. This type of hormonal treatment is not recommended for women with cancer or arteriosclerosis, however; at the very least, these patients must be monitored by a medical professional. Vaginal bleeding may occur on the days such treatment is discontinued; this could mean that the estradiol and progesterone doses were too high. When this happens, you should restart your hormones at half the dose that was prescribed during the previous cycle, consult a gynecologist, or stop treatment. The recommended doses are progesterone cream 20 milligrams twice a day, estradiol (Estrogel) 0.725 milligrams in the morning for 26 days with a 4-day break; DHEA 25 milligrams in the morning once a week; and T4 25 micrograms once a day increased to 50 micrograms while monitoring your body temperature.

The use of these two hormones together is essential to determine the ratio of progesterone to estradiol (the P/E2 ratio), which should be 50 or more. This ratio is important; studies have shown that if it is maintained, there is a good chance of preventing breast cancer and other types of cancer. A combination of the three hormones—estradiol, progesterone, and T3—will also cause weight loss and reduce total cholesterol and LDL cholesterol levels while increasing HDL (high-density lipoprotein). You will be advised to reduce your carbohydrate intake to reduce your triglyceride and cholesterol levels and control your blood pressure. The use of these two hormones together will also improve your energy and vitality, prevent depression and osteoporosis, and improve insulin activity while modulating blood sugar levels, while helping you relax to reduce stress and cortisol levels in the blood. They will also improve immune system activity. Patients experiencing sleep problems may take melatonin 10 milligrams before going to bed and perform physical activity between 5 pm and 6 pm to improve their sleep. This should be done until you can sleep continuously for 8 to 9 hours a day.

Case report

NAME OF TEST	RESULTS	NORMAL RANGE
Cholesterol	250.5 mg/dL	110(................)*200
LDL-Cholesterol	155.2 mg/dL	40(.................)*130
Estradiol	105 pmol/L	Less of 188
TSH	2.49 mIU/L	0.3(.........*.....)4.2
FT3	3.8 pmol/L	3.5(..*...........)6.5
FT4	13.8 pmol/L	10(.....*.........)20
DHEA	1.95 Umol/L	0.9(.*..............)11.6
Cortisol	484 nmol L	118(..........*...)690

Figure 8-9. Laboratory test results for a 59-year-old woman who complained of fatigue throughout the day, as well as urinary disturbances, fluid retention, high cholesterol (despite taking statins), and weight gain. Test results show an increase in cholesterol and LDL levels and low-normal levels of T3, T4, DHEA, and testosterone, which explains the fatigue and the increase in cholesterol. The estradiol level is high for her age and indicates the possibility of hormonal overcontrol of estradiol. The progesterone test was not performed. Abbreviations: DHEA, dehydroepiandrosterone; FT3, free triiodothyronine; FT4, free thyroxine; TSH, thyroid-stimulating hormone.

NAME OF TEST	RESULTS	NORMAL RANGE
Cholesterol	158 mg/dL	110(.......*........)200
Cholesterol LDL	89 mg/dL	40(....*.............)130
Estradiol	194 pmol/L	Less than 188
TSH	2.02 mIU/L	0.3(........*........)4.2
FT3	4.6 pmol/l	3.5(.........*........)6.5
FT4	16 pmol/L	10(........*........)20
DHEA	8.9 pmol/L	0.9(..........*.....)11.6
Cortisol	395 nmol/L	118(........*......)690
Progesterone	1.9	
P/E2 ratio	9.79	less than 50

Figure 8-10. These laboratory tests were taken after the patient described in Figure 8-9 had been treated with T4, DHEA (25 milligrams), and progesterone. The average values for cholesterol and LDL are included. The T3 and testosterone levels increased slightly, along with DHEA. The P/E ratio did not reach the desired level, however, then the progesterone dose should be increased. Abbreviations: DHEA, dehydroepiandrosterone; FT3, free triiodothyronine; FT4, free thyroxine; P/E, progesterone/estradiol ratio; TSH, thyroid stimulating hormone.

The patient received biological hormones as needed, as well as vitamin D, vitamin B, magnesium, and coenzyme Q10, and instructions for a healthy diet, along with instructions for physical activity according to her ability. For about 6 months, there was gradual improvement in her feelings, she slept well, and the fatigue decreased considerably. She stopped taking all of her usual medications, including the cholesterol-lowering medication; her blood test results were as shown in Figure 8-10 and include a decrease in cholesterol and LDL and improvement in the natural hormones. In this way, the lipid profile and the quality of life can be improved because the metabolic rate has increased, and the body has begun to use cholesterol for energy production.

In conclusion!

Over the past 30 years since I left the field of conventional medicine and stopped taking medication, I have come to understand many things and made many new discoveries. These discoveries about my body and what it needs to function properly have allowed me to live another 32 years in good health. This doesn't mean that I haven't aged, but the aging process has been easier for me than for others. Sometimes I don't feel like I'm aging at all compared with other people my age whom I see on the street. At my good old age of 85, I can go where I want without a cane or a walker and enjoy the view, enjoy life, and be creative. This book is a summary of the personal experiences I gained in treating women for various diseases over these many years. If any medical problem occurred, I would recognize it quickly. I would fix it because of the precise and accurate decoding of the lab test I created.

Overall, our health problems are the result of hormonal imbalances and a lack of vitamins and minerals. You need hormones like you need oxygen. As you already understand having read Chapter 1, the mitochondrion is the spring of life. If we take care of it, it will produce the energy and heat we need to live and allow us to take care of our health. The oxygen we get is free; it is the first thing we need to take care of our health. The mitochondria will function well over time, provided they get the hormones they need to refresh and renew their enzyme pools throughout the entire body. You have seen how we can take medicine and the mitochondria do not produce energy. As a result, we start to deteriorate. The same thing happened to me 30 years ago when I found out that I was being poisoned by all the drugs I was taking for high blood pressure, diabetes, high cholesterol levels, and cancer. My hormone levels were very low! The problem is yourself. You have health service insurance, yet you have passed the responsibility for your health entirely to your doctor, hoping he will cure your disease. But the drug companies want you to be constantly sick so that you will continue to use their drugs; they also want to confuse your doctor with a lot of wrong information. That's how I discovered the reason for my deteriorating health. I took drugs that did not cure me at all. The proof was that when I gave my body the hormones it needed to function, I lived another 30 years—and I think I could go on like this for a bit longer. Eventually we will have a cure for various diseases using natural hormones supplements.

That is why you must take responsibility for your health and understand what is going on in your body. If you don't help yourself, nobody will do it. That is the world in which you live.

Chapter 9

Hidden Hypothyroidism
and Pregnancy

Thyroid disease is common among women of childbearing age. Thyroid disorders may manifest for the first time during pregnancy. Because symptoms of thyroid disease can resemble those of pregnancy, the diagnosis can be challenging, especially when it is based on the TSH (thyroid-stimulating hormone) level alone. Many cases of hidden hypothyroidism are missed in women because they are pregnant or taking thyroxine (T4). The fetus depends on the mother for an adequate supply of T4 and triiodothyronine (T3). It is necessary to emphasize thyroid disorders in pregnant women so that appropriate treatment can be started as soon as possible to ensure optimal results. Proper, timely treatment can prevent complications during pregnancy and childbirth and reduce the incidence of congenital or neurological disorders in the fetus. Using the TSH level alone, the doctor could miss thyroid hypoactivity in pregnant patients. The World Health Organization (WHO) initiative to add iodine to table salt significantly reduced the incidence of hereditary hypothyroidism and disabilities in newborns, but the problem of low T3 levels in the general population still exists.

When a woman becomes pregnant, her thyroid gland activity increases by 50% to 75%, her T4 and T3 hormone levels rise, and her TSH is very low. Reduced 5'deiodinase (known as 5'D) activity—which results in a reduced T4/T3 conversion rate—may be the problem. This can occur if TSH levels drop significantly, which makes it challenging to diagnose hypoactivity. Although the fetus receives these hormones from the mother during the first 4 months of pregnancy, fetal thyroid hormone levels can still be less than optimal. Among other things, thyroid hormones enable normal fetal development, including the development of the nervous system and the rest of the body. A normal level of thyroid hormones provides the energy needed for fetal stem cells to divide and form a typical body structure and nervous system. An inadequate level of these hormones in the mother during the first few months of pregnancy may result in permanent damage to the fetus.

In this modern era, many children are born with neurological disorders and congenital disabilities that first show up at birth or during the early development of the child. These disorders include autism and attention-deficit/hyperactivity disorder (ADHD), which may disrupt their lives and the lives of their parents. This chapter is intended for the pregnant woman who wants to know whether her thyroid gland is functioning correctly before and during pregnancy so that her fetus can develop healthfully. Because the usual laboratory test decoding measures are not sensitive enough to diagnose hypothyroidism, I am providing herein some simple instructions she can use to put her mind at rest.

In conventional medicine, hypothyroidism is diagnosed according to TSH and T4 levels that are not within normal limits; doctors do not measure the T3 level or body temperature to make a more accurate diagnosis. If not, do the T3 test privately. This information may be necessary in cases of latent hypoactivity in women. A blood test may show a high TSH level (above 2 mIU/L). In that case, the standard treatment is to get the T4 level to its normal range. The T4/T3 conversion rate is not usually checked, however. If it is too low, the mother could develop complications during pregnancy and childbirth. To become pregnant, the woman must have an average body temperature of around 36.8 to 37.0 degrees Celsius (98.2-98.6 degrees Fahrenheit) during the day and an optimal level of progesterone (see Chapter 8). When she is already pregnant, the fetus requires T4 and T3. If the mother is stressed, smokes, or drinks alcohol, she loses some of her T3 values and the T4/T3 conversion rate is reduced. As a result, her T3 levels will not reach the upper third of the normal limit during her pregnancy. If she is experiencing latent thyroid hypoactivity (low T3 syndrome), the fetus may develop abnormally, even if she is taking T4 only. This situation may persist during the pregnancy and cause the fetus to develop a neurologic disorder, congenital disability, or any of several other diseases that are not always detected during a routine fetal echo study during pregnancy.

During the first 4 months of pregnancy, the fetus receives T4 and T3 from the mother through the placenta. Both mother and fetus need an additional 100 micrograms of iodine per day. The mother's T4 is the primary hormone reaching the fetus through the placenta. The placental 5'D level can convert it to T3 if her progesterone, estradiol, vitamin, and mineral levels are normal. The thyroid gland develops in the fetus after the fourth month of pregnancy. Does the placenta or the mother's 5'D convert enough T4 to T3 for the fetus? In any case, the mother usually needs more T3 to maintain the pregnancy and experience birth without complications. To be sure, T3, T4, and TSH laboratory tests can give you the answer according to the accurate decoder system described in this book, together with temperature measurements taken in the morning and mid-day. Hence, the importance of a correct and accurate diagnosis of thyroid gland function during the first 4 months of pregnancy and an optimal T3 level and progesterone/estradiol ratio will help avoid miscarriage or complications during pregnancy and birth.

Case Presentation: 34-year-old woman who has been unable to get pregnant for 5 years

Ronit, who is 34 years old, has been married 5 years but has been unable to get pregnant. She complains of symptoms of hypothyroidism and estradiol dominance (Figures 9-1 – 9-3).

NAME OF TEST	RESULTS	NORMAL RANGE
Estradiol	1110 pmol/L	72(................)*530
TSH	1.12 mIU/L	0.55(...*..........)4.78
Free T3	4.4 pmol/L	3.5(........*.......)6.5
Free T4	10.1 pmol/L	10(*................)20
LH	17.8 IU/L	0.5(..............)*16.9
FSH	5.9 IU/L	1.5(........*.........)9.1
Progesterone	<2 nmol/L	9*(.................)68
Cortisol	257 nmol/L	138(...*............)690

Figure 9-1. Hormonal lab values for Ronit. Her estradiol level is very high compared with her progesterone level, resulting in a P/E ratio of 1.8.(2.0 ÷ 1.110).

Her FT4 level is very low, and her FT3 level is relatively low, which suggests low T3 syndrome. Her temperature was 36.4 degrees Celsius (97.5 degrees Fahrenheit). Abbreviations: FSH, follicle-stimulating hormone; LH, luteinizing hormone; T3, triiodothyronine; T4, thyroxine; TSH, thyroid-stimulating hormone.

Her test results reveal estradiol dominance syndrome and hypothyroidism, which explains why she couldn't get pregnant. She was treated with progesterone, avoiding food that contains phytoestrogen, T3, and T4. Her laboratory results, taken 3 months after therapy began, appear in Figure 9-2.

NAME OF TEST	TEST RESULTS	NORMAL RANGE
Estradiol	467 pmol/	71(..........*...)530
TSH	0.07 mIU/L	0.55*(.............)4.78
Free T3	5.7 pmol/L	3.5(...........*...)6.5
Free T4	11.6 pmol/L	10(..*..............)20
Beta-hCG	< 5	---
Prolactin	118.5 mIU/L	138*(..............)690
Progesterone	49.3 nmol/L	9(............*...)68

Figure 9-2. Hormonal lab results for Ronit after 3 months of treatment with progesterone, T3, and T4. The relationship among the hormones is normal. P/E ratio: 49.2 ÷ 0.467=105. Her body temperature rose to the range of 36.8 to 37.0 degrees Celsius (98.2 – 98.6 degrees Fahrenheit). Abbreviations: hCG, human chorionic gonadotropin; T3, Triiodothyronine; T4, thyroxine; TSH, thyroid-stimulating hormone.

The condition in utero, the body temperature, and thyroid function were adequate for Ronit to become pregnant. I recommended that she and her husband take a short vacation.

NAME OF TEST	RESULTS	NORMAL RANGE
Estradiol	7677pmol/L	71(................)*530
Progesterone	92.90 nmol/L	9(................)*68
Beta hCG	76660	---

Figure 9-3. Ronit is pregnant.!! She continued to take T3 and T4 and progesterone throughout the pregnancy. The birth passed without complications. She came to my house to show me her baby.

This treatment—T4, T3, and progesterone—was used in five more young women, all of whom became pregnant.

Hypothyroidism Symptoms During Pregnancy

During pregnancy, many women complain of feeling tired; being overly sensitive to cold temperatures; and having a hoarse voice, facial swelling, abnormal weight gain, edema, constipation, obesity, gestational diabetes, high blood pressure, skin and hair changes, dry skin, and unusual muscle contractions. If a miscarriage or premature birth occurs, if the woman finds herself unable to concentrate, or other complaints arise, these are often attributed to the pregnancy itself.

Recent evidence shows that mild maternal thyroid underactivity during pregnancy may have a long-term effect on the child's cognitive development and carry a risk for neurodevelopmental disorders. Furthermore, these changes appear to be largely irreversible after birth if the mother or the infant's condition was not recognized before then.

The mother-to-be is usually expected to recover after birth. Imagine, however, if she had been under prolonged stress during pregnancy or had a prolonged or complicated birth involving heavy blood loss. Her cortisol level may have increased; as a result, the rate of T4/T3 conversion during pregnancy and after birth may have decreased. If so, the mother would remain in a state of latent thyroid hypoactivity. That is why she did not recover. She can't breastfeed the baby because of a lack of milk. She can't take care of her baby; she becomes depressed or refuses to receive her baby because of a lack of oxytocin (the "love hormone"). These are all signs of hypothyroidism that may persist after birth.

Case Presentation: 40-year-old women following a prolonged, complicated birth

Hana, who is 40 years old, gave birth to her second son one year ago. The birth was prolonged and complicated. Many months after giving birth, she had not recovered: She stopped lactating and had to feed her child powdered milk. She complained of severe fatigue that caused prolonged stress and lack of sleep. Her thyroid laboratory test results show the problem (Figure 9-4).

Name	Results	Units	Reference Range	Average Range
TSH	0.5	mIU/L	0.5-4.8	*..........
FT4	12.7	pmol/L	10.3-19.7	....*
FT3	4.56	pmol/L	3.5-6.5	......*......

Figure 9-4. Hana's postpartum thyroid hormone levels provide evidence of thyroid hypoactivity.

Figure 9-4 shows a very low TSH level (probably due to prolonged stress from giving birth until now). Her T4 level is below the midpoint. Her T3 level is also below the upper level—which would be expected, given that a very low TSH level indicates that there is not enough T3 to provide the energy she needs. The T4/T3 conversion rate is also low because stress interferes with

5'D activity. As a result, she is weak and unable to function.

Hana received the standard treatment of T4 50 micrograms and T3 50 micrograms to compensate for the amount of stress she had endured and the low T4/T3 conversion rate. Shortly thereafter, she recovered completely.

Chapter 10

Fibromyalgia

Fibromyalgia is a mysterious disease that brings the patient to the doctor with many complaints. Still, the doctor cannot make a diagnosis because of a lack of appropriate laboratory tests or imaging techniques that can be used to detect it. In the past, this was considered a psychiatric disease; most of the time, the patient was treated with psychiatric drugs. Recently, however, it was defined as a psychosomatic disease—one of those disorders in the functioning of the nervous system that leads to a disruption in the body's ability to function normally. After it was determined that the brain manages the activity of every cell in the body through hormones, it became clear that many patients go through a period of prolonged emotional stress before developing this disease, a period marked by disturbances in the activity of the hypothalamus—→adrenal gland—→thyroid axis.

Fibromyalgia also coexists with other diseases that are characterized by an inflammatory process involving the whole body, such as autoimmune, viral, or drug-induced diseases in which cortisol levels are high. A patient who is in a state of chronic stress, anxiety, or depression may develop a hormonal imbalance and sleep disturbances as a result of an increase in cortisol secretion. Many glands demonstrate abnormalities that are manifested in various ways on laboratory tests—for example, a lack of serotonin, and increase in platelets volume, as well as hypothyroidism or low magnesium levels—and as severe menstrual disorders, migraine headaches, sleep disorders, and food allergies. In the past, these conditions appeared in patients who had had repeated episodes of stress or depression.

Symptoms of fibromyalgia

Fibromyalgia is characterized by prolonged muscle and joint pain without local inflammatory signs. Women are more likely to experience it than men, exhibiting chronic fatigue, sleep disorders, mood changes (depression or anxiety), difficulty concentrating, memory disorders, confused and disorganized thoughts, migraines, and premenstrual syndrome. The body temperature usually remains lower than 36.8 degrees Celsius (98.2 degrees Fahrenheit). In all, these symptoms lead to disturbances in sexual and digestive functions, along with a change in weight. Patients with fibromyalgia exhibit various urinary disorders, including recurrent urinary tract infections. All of these symptoms can change from day to day to the point of becoming daily functional disorders. What characterizes the disease, however, is the hypersensitivity of muscles and joints in some regions of the body to touch.

What are the reasons for the development of this disease?

The laboratory picture for these patients is complex. Their cortisol levels are in the upper half of the average value instead of the lower half, where it should be. Because a red asterisk is not associated with it, the doctor refers to it as "an expected result." Some patients with fibromyalgia also experience chronic fatigue syndrome with low cortisol levels because the adrenal gland is exhausted. Due to prolonged stress, the asterisk will appear in the lower third of the normal range after the adrenal gland has stopped functioning. As we learned in previous chapters, a high cortisol level leads to a hormonal imbalance—a decrease in DHEA, IGF-1, T3, testosterone, and progesterone and an increase in estradiol. As a result, several disorders develop in a woman's menstrual cycle and in male fertility. Because it involves a permanent inflammatory state, fibromyalgia is marked by elevated levels of cytokines (small proteins that trigger immune activity) and C-reactive protein (CRP; a plasma protein that increases in concentration in response to inflammation), and allergic reactions abound. As we learned in previous chapters, these proteins affect the hypothalamus function and cause the hormonal imbalance in the body. Patients with this disorder also experience mood disorders and marked changes in the serotonin and dopamine levels in the brain that may explain the bouts of depression and anxiety and the lack of sleep (low levels of serotonin cause sleep disturbances and depression; high levels of serotonin cause mental restlessness and anxiety attacks). Along with depression, decreased serotonin levels in the brain, and hormonal imbalances, many patients with this condition become addicted to carbohydrates and, consequently, gain weight. Doctors usually administer medications targeting each symptom.

Mitochondrial dysfunction was found to develop in patients with fibromyalgia because of multiple nutritional deficiencies.

As a result, the body does not produce enough energy to keep the cells in the body functioning properly. It was even found that patients with this disorder may have a deficiency in coenzyme Q10 and other components of the mitochondria that are essential to create energy particles (ATPs; see Chapter 1) in the cells. High levels of free radicals have also been found in these patients. If this is not enough, about 5 years ago, a patient with fibromyalgia exhibited a high level of immunoglobulin E (IgE) antigens due to allergies to various foods (see later). Blood tests for IgE allergies showed that she was sensitive to milk, gluten, vitamin C, shaving cream, and other substances. Practitioners of conventional medicine do not have the tools to treat allergies. I recommended that a patient who develops such allergies find a practitioner of Chinese medicine to follow the method used by Dr. Nambudripad Devi (the NEAT approach) to eliminate them. Her allergic reactions had caused muscle pain, fatigue, and joint pain, as well as a runny nose, itching, diarrhea, and various types of skin rashes, among other reactions. After these were eliminated, she felt significant relief. All of the systems affected in this patient are managed by the hippocampus, which warns the body about toxic substances in food or in the environment that originate through the industrial or agricultural treatment of expensive milks and meats. The patient now checks every food item to determine if there is any potential for sensitivity. In this way, you too can avoid many allergy symptoms. Please look for professional information about this technique for getting rid of fibromyalgia-associated food allergies while balancing your hormones.

What You Can Do If You Develop Fibromyalgia

All of your laboratory test results will probably be considered "normal." Photographs or imaging study results will also be "normal" according to conventional medicine's guidelines. In other words, the asterisk on the test report will be within the normal range of average values. When fibromyalgia appears in the context of other diseases with positive laboratory tests, however, the doctor will concentrate on treating the new condition according to his field of expertise. By contrast, practitioners of functional medicine see the body as one unit and will interpret your laboratory test results more accurately using the decoding rules presented in this book. If you develop fibromyalgia, you should ask the doctor to conduct a hormonal investigation by running the following laboratory tests: anti-thyroid peroxidase (anti-TPO) antigen and antithyroglobulin (anti-TG) antibody, TSH, free T3 (FT3), free T4 (FT4), cortisol, DHEA, minerals, vitamins, iron, estradiol, progesterone, testosterone, and vitamin D (Figure 10-2).

Test Name	Results	Units	Reference Vakue	Range Value
Magnesium	1	mg/dl	1.9-2.5	*............
Vitamin B12	368	pg/m l	211-911	....*.........
Protein Total	6.4	g/dl	6.6-8.3	*..............
WBC Leucocytes	4.1	10.*3	4.5-11	*.............
MCV	90	FL	80-98	.............*..
RBC	4.41	10*6	-52	*.............
Hemoglobin	13	g/dl	12.5-16	*.............
Hematocrit	46	%	36-46	.............*
TSH	6.39	IU/ml	0.64-5.5	.............*
TPO Ag's	42.2	IU/ml	0-60	..........*......

Abbreviations: DHEA, dehydroepiandrosterone; Mg, magnesium; MPV, mean platelet volume; P/E2 ratio, progesterone/estradiol ratio; RBC, red blood cells; T3, triiodothyronine; WBC, white blood cells.

Figure 10-2. Laboratory test findings in fibromyalgia.

Interpreting these test results using my approach, you can see signs of nutritional deficiency: the magnesium, iron, vitamin C, and ferritin (iron stores) levels are very low due to severe disturbances in the intestinal absorption. It is also apparent that the mitochondria are not producing enough energy, as indicated by the very low levels of vitamin B12, vitamin B1, copper, testosterone, DHEA, T3, and proteins. There is also a low number of platelets within a large volume—this is typical of fibromyalgia, but also hypothyroidism, given that both T3 and T4 are at their lowest levels within the acceptable range. The cortisol level is also low, reflecting the chronic fatigue syndrome associated with adrenal exhaustion due to prolonged stress. The previous report also indicates estradiol dominance, for which the patient is receiving progesterone. Her P/E2 ratio is more than 50, because the test was done while she was taking progesterone. Her immune system is weak, however, as indicated by a low level of vitamin D and the low number of white blood cells (mainly neutrophils and lymphocytes).

These test results are puzzling to the attending physician, because most of the asterisks are within the average normal range. That could make it difficult to diagnose this disease.

How this patient was treated

The patient was given the following advice:

1. **Reduce stress.** This is a difficult task, because modern life always presents us with enough stress to make complete healing difficult. Women who have experienced complex events and soldiers who have experienced depression after wartime trauma may need help from a professional psychotherapist who can teach them how to practice meditation. They should also be given hormone replacement therapy with biological hormones that are 100% identical to the substances produced by the body: T3, 50 micrograms; DHEA, 25 micrograms; vitamin D, 5000 International Units, and progesterone, 40 milligrams; plus multivitamins, calcium, iron, and magnesium while following a Paleo diet. You can eat a few pieces of chocolate.

2. **Improve sleep.** Sometimes we can't sleep because the events of the past come to mind, even at night. This causes stress to remain throughout the night. Sleeping pills may fail to silence these negative thoughts, which may result in the need for a sedative, such as Valium®. Unfortunately, this can lead to addiction. To control negative thoughts at night, as well as during the day, I recommend learning meditation techniques, such as the Barry Long method. It might

be helpful to take melatonin for sleep and GABA 750 milligrams to relax and reduce muscle pain. Physical activity, like walking for half an hour at 5 pm, can also help you sleep. In any treatment with natural hormones, we need to find the dose that suits us. The goal is to sleep continuously for 8 to 9 hours.

3. **Get your allergies treated.** Many patients with fibromyalgia are sensitive to a particular food—milk and milk products, wheat, eggs, sugar, alcohol, or spices—or nutrient—vitamin B, C, or D, as well as calcium and certain proteins—or substances in the environment, including mold, Candida organisms, worms, industrial materials, laundry softener, and chemicals used in the home. From my experience, Chinese medicine is an excellent approach to getting rid of allergies. It can also help you get rid of the pain in the muscles and joints that occur because of this disease.

4. **Treat an underactive thyroid gland.** T3 should be added to your therapeutic routine while your temperature is being monitored. It is possible that T4 is not being converted to T3 because of the inflammatory condition in your body.

Chapter 11

Attention Deficit Disorder (ADD) and Hyperactivity Disorder (ADHD)

This chapter is dedicated to my family members, particularly my grandchildren and their mothers, who told me about the difficulties they go through when a child is found to have an attention disorder. I use my common sense and experience to take care of these children. This is how I treated my own child intuitively when he was small and hyperactive. Some of my grandchildren also have attention deficit/hyperactivity disorder (ADHD), but their treatment is the responsibility of the parents; I can only advise them. These illnesses are described in about 7% of the children in Israel. The syndrome is diagnosed during kindergarten or later when the child does not follow the teacher's instructions or seems nervous, restless, or unfocused or is violent toward other children.

There is no effective medical treatment for this syndrome. Approximately 5% to 10% of the world's population is believed to have ADHD or attention-deficit disorder (ADD) lasting into their old age (there are estimates that this affects as much as 20% of the population). My impression is that the number is actually higher, because many people show mental disturbances later in life that were not diagnosed. For every girl with ADD or ADHD, there are three to five boys with the syndrome. Sometimes it is accompanied by autism. There is a belief that it is inherited, but it is also assumed that it is the result of a lack of various biological components in the mother during pregnancy—mainly underactivity of the thyroid gland that was not diagnosed by general medicine practitioners with the usual decoding approach.

The mother complained about it during pregnancy (see the discussion of hypoactivity in Chapter 9) or while breastfeeding. But all of her laboratory test results were "normal," because they were based on a TSH and T4 test only. This condition prevents normal brain development in the fetus or in the baby and may also affect the child's genes. This possibility probably exists in light of the latest scientific findings, which show that food can change attitude in 60% of children with ADHD/ADD. Many of them continue to show various signs of the syndrome even into adulthood, however.

The causes of ADD/ADHD are related to hereditary, as well as environmental and nutritional influences on the mother. First, it should be noted that for the brain to develop properly from the embryonic period until adolescence, the following biological substances are needed:

1. Proteins, especially those with the amino acids phenylalanine, tryptophan, tyrosine, and L-glutamine.

2. The B vitamins, as well as vitamins C and E and folic acid; and the minerals iron, zinc, magnesium, copper, manganese, and iodine.

3. Calorigenic nutrients, including essential fatty acids (such as omega-3), cholesterol, and complex carbohydrates, including those that supply the essential polysaccharides that are found in breast milk and food.

A deficiency in one or more of these biological substances has been found in children with ADHD and autism. Nobody is considering this problem as an endocrine problem of the thyroid gland.

I think all of these conclusions are confusing. The root of the problem in ADHD/ADD is the lack of energy (due to a low of T3 blood levels) during the baby's developmental stages. This can lead to a defensive shunt that will accompany him for life. I intended to check the temperature in children with autism or Down syndrome, but I was blocked by the institution manager. I present the case of an adult with ADHD in Chapter 6. The mother's eating habits and smoking because of stress also had an effect in her hormonal balance.

Symptoms of ADHD and ADD

I suggest you learn to identify the symptoms of this disorder in a young child and follow its development as the child grows older. If your child shows these symptoms as a baby or when he starts walking, it is possible to help his brain continue its development so that he can become a normal child. Measure his body temperature orally for a minute in the morning when he wakes up; it should be 36.5 degrees Celsius or higher. By midday, before lunch, it should be 36.9 to 37 degrees. If it does not rise until noon, he will be restless. If his temperature is low in the morning, he may appear hyperkinetic as his body tries to increase the flow of blood and energy to his brain. Ask your doctor to measure his TSH, T4, and T3 levels. Perhaps he is under stress. An 8 am cortisol test reading should be in the middle or high range of normal values; this test should be interpreted as I have explained elsewhere in this book. His T3 level should be at the top of the normal curve, and his T4 level should be in the middle. A high T3 level is necessary to permit normal brain and body development. If necessary, you can give him 25 micrograms of T4 until his temperature returns to normal (around 37 degrees Celsius during the day). Don't worry: This treatment does not cause the thyroid gland to atrophy. It is possible to take breaks from the T4 treatment for a week to watch the child's conduct with and without T4 therapy and a healthy diet (i.e., a week or two during which industrial fats like canola oil are not used for cooking, dairy products or even organic dairy products [these have much fewer trans fats than regular milk and milk products] diet are only used on during these days, and fast foods are avoided). Other weeks without T4 and permits regular diet. Support the child and help him carry out some physical activities. Start the program by giving him T4 to keep his temperature up, and he will be quiet. Over time, he will get used to doing physical activities regularly because it will calm him down and it is socially accepted. As a result, he may have more friends to play with, which will boost his self-esteem.

The signs of ADHD are (1) motor problems associated with overactivity; (2) attention problems; (3) various psychiatric disorders, aggressive or violent behavior, and excessive talking; (4) addiction to candies or condiments; and (5) isolation (see case report in Chapter 6).

All of these symptoms are characterized by a persistent pattern of inattention and/or hyperactivity and impulsivity appearing more frequently and in a more severe form compared with children who are characterized by their peers as having an appropriate and quiet motor activity.

These children instinctively increase blood flow to the brain by increasing their own physical activity to generate more energy in it.

The following phenomena have been observed in children with motor disorders:

1. Restlessness and twisting of their arms and legs while sitting in a chair.
2. Inability to stay still or sit still.
3. Inability to find space in his environment for other children.
4. Excessive talking.
5. Losing his ability to concentrate visually, quickly switching from one TV program to another or having difficulty reading and understanding a book.
6. Difficulty functioning in leisure activities.
7. Problems paying attention.

These children show antisocial behaviors that may affect them later in life, including the following:

1. Difficulty waiting for service in line.
2. Chronic lateness and laziness.
3. Compulsive and continuous talking without giving other children the opportunity to speak.
4. Difficulty starting or finishing tasks.
5. Reading problems and low academic achievement because of difficulty concentrating. Apparently, this problem is also related to the child's inability to focus his eyes on the text he is reading.
6. Dependence on a rigid regimen to function.
7. Noticeable lack of organization and lack of attention to details.

Mood disorders

One set of the prominent phenomena that parents have to deal with in their children's behavior consists of unexplained mood disorders, such as the following:

8. Fits of anger.
9. Detachment and lack of concern about what is happening around them.
10. Inappropriate behavior in social gatherings.
11. Anxiety and depression.
12. A feeling of hopelessness.

Addiction and alienation

Adults and older children with ADHD/ADD can easily reach various states of addiction and exhibit abnormal behaviors associated with addiction at an older age:

1. Addiction to drugs, carbohydrates, and sweets.
2. Smoking.
3. Excessive intake of alcohol.
4. Violence against others and crime.
5. Difficulty or inability to maintain relationships and intimacy with others.

Diagnosis

A diagnosis of ADHD/ADD is made by a pediatrician using special tests that consist of several components:

1. Exhibition of six or more symptoms from the list in Diagnostic and Statistical Manual of Mental Disorders, Edition IV to confirm the diagnosis.
2. Persistence of these symptoms for at least 6 months with a severity that does not correspond with the child's level of development.
3. Neurological examination to rule out underlying diseases.
4. Psychological test.
5. Didactic test.

Differential diagnosis with similar disorders
Other possible explanations for the child's behavior must be taken into account. For example:
1. Posttraumatic stress disorder: Children who have experienced emotional, physical, or sexual trauma show signs of defensiveness and hypervigilance.
2. Bipolar syndrome. These children experience the results of conflicts between their parents and/or between themselves and their parents and may have an excessive preoccupation with sex (verbal or practical) and an inflated sense of self-esteem.

Do you know this baby? Parents may notice abnormal phenomena in their baby's behavior during the early stages of his life. Many babies with ADHD exhibit allergic symptoms or the following:
1. Sleep disorder and eating disorder.
2. Stuffy or runny nose.
3. Stool that is too hard or too soft.
4. Heavy secretion of saliva and sweat.
5. Red and burning cheeks.
6. Recurring ear infections or fluid in the ears.
7. Screaming too much.
8. Makes it difficult to hold in your arms but likes to be bounced.
9. Walking early.

These signs are not necessarily related to ADHD, but children who exhibit them should be monitored. Take your child's temperature by mouth to test in a real situation and get the doctor's attention.

Do you know this toddler? Between the ages of one and 6 years, the following symptoms may appear:

1. Hyperactivity: a tendency to exhibit tantrums, biting, hitting, or spitting.
2. Leg pain, headaches, swollen stomach due to indigestion, stuffy nose, or ear infections. All of these are allergic reactions, usually to food.

Do you know this boy? In pre-compulsory or compulsory kindergarten, the teacher notices unusual phenomena in the child, such as the following:
1. Being hyperactive or easily irritated, exhibiting tantrums and behavior disorders.
2. Being tired or sad, staying by himself, preferring to be alone
3. Exhibiting allergic reactions: stuffy nose, cough, shortness of breath (asthma), or swollen stomach.
4. Exhibiting difficulty learning or writing.

Awareness of motor disorders and attention or mood disorders usually arises when the child reaches the age of compulsory preschool or regular school, because he is required to sit down and concentrate on his studies.

Do you know this teenager? The following signs of ADHD/ADD appear in children aged 10 years and older:
1. Depression and fatigue.
2. Inability to stay quiet, but no longer hyperactive.
3. Acute mood swings.
4. Difficulty concentrating and remembering during his studies or at work.
5. Adjustment problems at work.
6. Inability to control anger.
7. Easily inclined to use drugs, smoke or other addicting substances.
8. Unable to organize tasks.
9. Chronically bored.

10. Frequent headaches, indigestion, hay fever, asthma, and muscle pain.

The parents of pre-military–aged boys face issues of addiction and alienation more frequently than parents of other children in this age group, as stated in the text.

Factors associated with ADD/ADHD

According to practitioners of general medicine, the main reason for the development of ADD/ADHD is unknown. Mothers of these children are tested to determine whether they have a hypoactive thyroid based on a TSH study only. In most cases, they are not tested according to the more accurate criteria using FT4 and FT3. Possible causes have been published, but everything that has been published confuses doctors and does not direct them to check the endocrine status of the mother correctly during pregnancy or the child, which is a critical period for the baby. Therefore, the onset of the disease is attributed to the factors I mentioned earlier.

A considerable amount of energy is needed for stem cells in the brain to develop properly and form effective electrical connections. Nerve cells in the brain must be covered by a myelin sheath—a "fatty coat"—to transmit electrical impulses efficiently. The most important source of this energy is glucose. If fewer of these protein conductors are produced in any area in the brain or in the whole brain, it means that less sugar is being consumed; therefore, the metabolism of the brain is decreased. In patients with ADHD, low consumption of sugar in the brain can be seen on a PET scan (also known as a positron emission tomography scan). Figure 11-1 shows the PET scan of an individual with ADHD and an individual without ADHD. Figure 11-2 showed a student with difficulty concentrating because he presents with deep defect in the frontal area of the brain. Areas of dysfunction, which are the result of the poor utilization of sugar, are indicated by the lack of a change in color. Sugar (glucose) is normally converted into energy by T3. Because of the poor utilization of sugar in these areas, neurotransmitters such as dopamine and others cannot be produced normally. As a result, the child loses his ability to concentrate and loses his long-term memory, which results in a change in activity and behavioral characteristics. Reduced dopamine activity in the frontal (anterior) and prefrontal (lateral frontal) areas of the brain are associated with low and ineffective performance in school subjects/activities that involve memory-related tasks. The temporal lobe, which is located in the area of the brain around the ears, helps us understand the words we hear and "see." The temporal lobe is also connected to the hypothalamus (see Chapter 2), which regulates certain metabolic processes and secretes certain neurohormones—releasing hormones or hypothalamic hormones—which, in turn, stimulate or inhibit the secretion of hormones from the pituitary gland. Thus, the hypothalamus controls body temperature, hunger, important aspects of parenting and maternal attachment behaviors, as well as thirst, fatigue, sleep, and circadian rhythms.

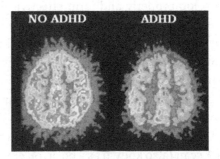

Figure 11-1. Left: PET scan of the brain of an individual without ADHD showing normal brain activity that is manifested because of appropriate sugar consumption. Right: PET scan of the brain of a child with ADHD. The image is taken from an article by Dr. Zadetkin et al. Abbreviations: ADHD, attention-deficit/hyperactivity disorder; PET, positron emission tomography.

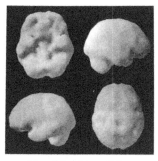
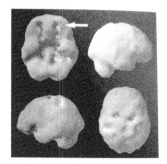

Overall healthy activity   Decreased prefrontal cortex activity

Figure 11-2. Left image Normal Right image during a reading exercise the upper left image (arrow) shows a deep and defective frontal area and concentration difficulties as well as minor defects in other areas.
(Taken from Daniel Amen Change Your Brain Change Your Body Book)

Researchers claim that there is a delay in the development of certain parts of the brain in children with ADHD. These include the prefrontal area, which, when damaged, causes inattention, hyperkinesis, and impulsivity; and the temporal area, which is responsible for our ability to concentrate. These findings suggest that children with ADHD probably lack important biological components (such as ATP; see Chapter 1) that are needed for normal brain development. They may lack these components because the mother had hypothyroidism or hidden thyroid underactivity that was not identified using the usual laboratory tests.

A Conventional Treatment: Ritalin®

The most common treatments for ADHD are stimulants: Ritalin® (methylphenidate), Concerta® (slow-release methylphenidate), Dexadrine® (dextroamphetamine), Desoxyl® (methamphetamine), Cylert® (pemoline), and Adderall® (mixed amphetamine salts). Ritalin, like other stimulants, stimulates brain activity by increasing the amount of dopamine and nor-epinephrine in the synapses in the brain, thereby improving motivation and cognitive functions in the patient. It does not treat the root of the problem, however: a low level of energy particles to use glucose in the brain.

Results of Ritalin treatment
In the short term, Ritalin is effective in reducing hyperactivity, recklessness, inattention, aggressiveness, and low academic achievements. It also eliminates any spontaneous activity by the child in games and in society and, thus, reduces their curiosity. In the long term, however, Ritalin does not result in any significant improvement in the patient's ability to achieve other milestones in life—for example, finishing 12 years of schooling, finding a permanent job, avoiding the use of drugs or alcohol, avoiding criminal acts—compared with other drugs used in this patient population.

"Mild" side effects of Ritalin
- The following side effects of Ritalin are defined as "mild":
- Loss of appetite
- Reduced growth rate due to decreased secretion of GH and IGF-1. These children are shorter than other children in the same age group
- Nausea and headaches
- Addictions
- Sleep disorders: Children with ADHD/ADD do not produce enough melatonin; therefore, they do not achieve a deep sleep (stage 4, or rapid eye movement sleep). They do not secrete enough GH, either and, thus, do not get enough sleep. As a result, they have difficulty waking up and are tired during the day

- Decreased ability to concentrate (related to stimulant effects of drug)
- Worsening of behaviors at the end of the drug's effective time

Serious side effects of Ritalin

According to the US Food and Drug Administration (FDA), instructions for the use of this drug must indicate that it may cause psychiatric events, which include "hallucinations, suicidal thoughts, psychotic behavior, violent and hostile behavior." The FDA also recommends adding a warning about the risk for sudden death and disturbances in heart activity. There have been 25 premature deaths among Americans who took these drugs. When the child has epileptic seizures, his condition is most likely related to hypothyroidism (See case report in this Chapter).

Complementary treatments

As you know, there is a connection between body and mind; therefore, psychological treatment can help calm the child with ADHD/ADD. Many methods are available to deal with the issue, but the treatment should be carried out by a qualified person who can direct the child according to his will. When you diagnose occult hypothyroidism early in the child's life, the child will be normal. The child will be disciplined and will appreciate the authority of the therapist. The psychological treatment of children with ADHD should be based on the following principles:

- A fixed and precise time and place for the activity
- Making direct eye contact with the child while talking to him
- Helping the child meditate, preferably at the beginning of the selected activity
- Using "Brain Gym" to improve the transfer of stimuli from

the left brain to the right brain and vice versa and coordinate activity between the right and left brain

- Using eye exercises to improve eye coordination in the child and help him focus better
- Convincing the child to take part in organized sports (for example: basketball, football, running, or swimming) as a means of using his hyperactivity to achieve relaxation, greater self-esteem, and strengthen his personality
- Healing in motion
- A healthy environment and a supportive and sympathetic attitude on the part of the parents and others
- Daily physical activity—a group basketball or tennis game or any other sport the child identifies with

If laboratory tests confirm ADHD/ADD according to the criteria presented here, start treatment with the T4 hormone at a dose of 25 micrograms and monitor the child's temperature and laboratory test results.

Case Report

A.Z. is an 11-year-old girl who was brought to me by her grandmother, who was concerned because the child lies in bed all day, is tired, does not interact with her classmates, and has low school results. This happened after her father, whom she loved, suddenly left home. One week later, she lost consciousness at school and was taken to a regional hospital, where she was diagnosed with epilepsy. She started taking anti-epileptic medications, which worsened her condition. The results of laboratory tests carried out by the attending physician were defined as "normal" (Figure 11-2). Her temperature was 36.2 degrees Celsius in the morning and 36.4 degrees at mid-day.

Test Name	Results	Units	Reference Values	Normal Range
TSH	0.65	uIU/dl	0.64-5.5	*............
ATP Abs	42.2	IU/ml	0-60.	..........*.....
ESR	0.6	mm/hr	0-20	...*.........

Figure 11-2. The TSH was very low, and the TPO Ag (42.2) was positive (the result must be zero!). I made a diagnosis of Hashimoto's thyroiditis and requested an FT3 test.

Name	Results	Units	Reference Range	Average Range
FT4	0.86	ng/dL	0.80-1.90	*.........
FT3	2.2	ng/dL	2.2-4.4	*.........
TSH	1.02	mIU/Ml	0.270-4.200	..*.........

Figure 11-3. TSH, FT3, and FT4 test results show a low level of each hormone in the patient's blood due to the anti-epileptic medication?

The patient started taking T4 25 micrograms and vitamins and was put on a gluten-free and protein diet. After one month, her mother reported that her body temperature had risen to 36.7 degrees and that she felt better and had returned to school. The neurologist refused to stop the anti-epileptic medication (Figure 11-3), even though the lab test showed a reduction in TSH, T4, and T3 levels because of the anti-epileptic drugs.

Name	Value	Units	Reference value	Range
FT4	0.87	pmo/L	0.8-1.9	*...........
FT3	3.5	pmo/L	2.0-4.4	........*....
TSH	0.855	pmo/L	0.270-4.20	*............

Figure 11-4. These results show improvement in FT3, but the T4 is still low. I increased The T4 to 50 micrograms.

Good nutrition

Diet is a very important element in the treatment of this child. As you saw earlier, her diet must consist of high-quality proteins and natural nutritious ingredients that help the brain develop properly from an early age. Trans fats should be avoided, especially from dairy products. Every 100 grams contain 0.5 grams to 0.8 grams of trans fat, mainly from the yolk of the egg, canola oil, margarine butter, and others. These products increase allergic symptoms, thereby triggering the release of substances that can block T3 and T4 hormone receptors on the cell membranes. That is why many children with ADHD have a runny nose, asthma, skin rash, and other symptoms of a food allergy. Parents should help their child by preparing appropriate foods for them to take to school and to other activities. The following measures should be taken:

1. We live in a very toxic environment!! Avoid, as much as possible, industrially processed food and drinks for your children, because these foods do not contain vitamins!!! It is very important to look at the label of the product you are considering for your child and notice what is written in the symbol of the letter E (various chemical substances), looking for trans fats that causes of hypothyroidism. Your child's brain and body need these hormones to create energy and use sugar in the brain. There is nothing to do: You have to eat organic food that contains very little trans-fat and prepare

cakes and snacks at home. You will see your child behaving differently and being quieter.

2. Avoid food coloring, caramel and starch, and read the food labels to make sure the food does not contain any artificial flavors, fragrances, preservatives, or stabilizers, especially in yellow and red candies

3. Avoid drinking Coca-Cola, Orangeade, and other carbonated drinks and artificially colored sweets. Instead, drink orange juice and grape juice without chemical additives

4. Avoid simple carbohydrates, especially cakes, cookies, and any pastries that contain margarine, etc. The parents may need to make such snacks at home

5. Eat three meals a day consisting mainly of proteins, vegetables, and complex carbohydrates (brown rice, whole wheat without gluten, oats [contain PUFA fats!]), as well as tomatoes, barley, carrots, vegetables, champignon mushrooms, salmon, high-quality fats (olive oil, avocado,), and fruits

6. Take supplements. Children with ADD/ADHD often are deficient in vitamins, minerals, essential fatty acids, and proteins that are essential for the creation of chemical conductors between brain cells. Make sure the following nutritional supplements are provided (they can be added to water with lemon or orange juice or given in the form of candy):

   • Essential amino acids, which are found in a hydrophilic collagen protein powder product that dissolves in water.

   • Vitamin and mineral supplements for children that include the B vitamins as well as vitamins A, D, and E.

   • Herbs or GABA capsules to curb hyperactivity and moderate other excessive reactions.

   • Phosphatidyl serine to increase levels of the neurotransmitter acetylcholine and other neurotransmitters.

   • Omega 3 oils, supplied in capsules or omega-3-rich foods such as salmon or green tea to overcome allergic symptoms

The correct food choices are important. Meals should consist mainly of natural food choices of proteins (meat, poultry, turkey, fish), as well as greens, fresh fruits, and complex carbohydrates. Simple carbohydrates cause a sharp increase and decrease in sugar and insulin levels in the blood; about 2 hours after a high-carbohydrate meal, the child will start feeling restless due to hunger as a result of an imbalance of neurotransmitters in the brain.

Ritalin may achieve immediate and rapid results, especially in children with ADHD. The schoolteacher demands that the child remain quiet in the classroom. Over time, however, you do not help the child by giving him Ritalin, because most of the children who take it will continue to exhibit symptoms of this syndrome while going the wrong way.

Chapter 12

How You Can Identify ADHD in Adults

Symptoms of ADHD in adults

- Being a workaholic
- Feeling uncomfortable when sitting in meetings
- Reluctance to wait in line for service
- A love of excessive speed while driving
- Talking too much
- Talking while waiting in line
- Making inappropriate comments
- Talking a lot about friends on the cell phone or in meetings
- Inability to tolerate low stimulation
- Environmental dependence
- Delaying or postponing an action
- Inability to make a forced physical effort
- Sensitivity to the mood or suffering of others
- Lack of motivation
- Outbursts of rage for no apparent reason
- Social skills: incompetent or lacking social judgment

- Impatient over regular events in his or her life, becoming frustrated and wanting to do the job immediately
- Uncontrolled sleep, as well as eating, physical activity, and not to taking care about his health (for example, eating too many carbs and not exercising)
- Reluctance to wait for the computer to find the file he is searching for

Such wild behavior could lead to negative social reactions from his friends or his boss and occupational deficiencies. But maturity and aging may give you the insight required to neutralize your reactions and adjust your behavior accordingly. Some people with this disorder have difficulty finishing school, and this may result in a serious family conflict. Wisdom and age may also bring the insight that the impact of ADHD can be minimized by adjusting the environment to be friendly to the person with ADHD and by strategically structuring it to help him deal with his impulses. For example: A child who felt restless and frustrated sitting in class all day may feel much better with a career such as a real estate agent or working from home. During childhood, there may have been no regard for his problems; he just had to keep quiet and do what his parents told him to do. Today, parents are always welcome to speak with their child's teacher in school and receive warnings about the child's behavior from his teachers regarding any need to restrain the child's compulsive behaviors. Many children remain undiagnosed, however. The parents may also oppose the child's activities at home. The child's doctor may very quickly or automatically prescribe Ritalin® to control the child's behavior without first checking for physical signs of any cause of that behavior, such as low body temperature or low energy level (due, for example, to an inadequate output of T3). As adults, such individuals are not always able to control their behavior regarding diet and social relationships. Many prefer being alone, avoid physical activity, and do not take care of their health. If this sounds like you and your parents support you, you can start curbing your reactions and adjusting your reactions to work and family and control compulsive eating behaviors. If you understand what is going on in your brain and start taking T4 and T3, your brain might function properly. Most people with ADHD are highly intelligent, but that does not matter, given their social conduct and bad social connections. (Figure 12-1)

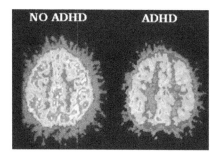

Figure 12-1. left, a normal adult brain; right, brain in an adult with ADHD.

While writing this book, I asked what happens to adults with ADHD who have taken Ritalin since childhood. I reviewed 11 articles that included responses from 475 individuals. In some of these studies, the investigators reported that immediate-release Ritalin reduced depression and anxiety; others reported no change, and still others described an increase in symptoms of depression and anxiety. The most common side effect was loss of appetite, which, in some cases, was accompanied by weight loss. In none of these studies were any of these effects reported as problematic or serious. These studies were short, however; therefore, their clinical significance could not be properly assessed. In five studies, investigators reported changes in systolic or diastolic blood pressure with Ritalin, and in three they reported an increase in heart rate. None of these results were considered a cause for concern. None of the studies reported any clinically significant side effects—cardiovascular or otherwise. In three studies, side effects were not even mentioned.

The condition of the thyroid gland was not properly checked in any of these studies. It is possible that they tested thyroid function using TSH only or looked for a red asterisk. If so, that is not enough. Put your brain in your hands; change your life with a brilliant brain taking T3.

LIST OF TERMS

5'Deiodinase	An enzyme responsible for the conversion of the T4 hormone to the T3 hormone; also known as 5D
ACTH	Hormone secreted by the pituitary gland; activates the adrenal gland to produce cortisol; also known as adrenocorticotropic hormone
Adrenal gland	One of a pair of small glands located just above the kidneys that secretes the hormones DHEA, cortisol, and aldosterone
Adrenaline	A hormone secreted by the adrenal gland to trigger visceral response to stress
Aldosterone	A hormone secreted by the adrenal gland to help maintain the water-salt balance in the body
Andropause	The middle age of the man
ATP	A molecule produced in the mitochondria that stores energy that will be used by the cell; also known as adenosine triphosphate
B vitamins	An important group of vitamins that supports normal enzymatic activity
BRCA1	A gene that is responsible for correcting gene mutations in breast tissue
BRCA2	A gene that is responsible for correcting gene mutations in breast tissue
Calcitonin	A hormone secreted by the thyroid gland to facilitate the absorption of calcium and magnesium from the intestines
Coenzyme Q10	A hormone that is secreted by the adrenal gland to regulate the body's response to stress
Cortisol	A hormone that is secreted by the adrenal gland to regulate the body's response to stress
CRP	A substance used to determine whether any inflammatory conditions exist in the body; also known as C-reactive protein.
DHEA	A hormone produced in the adrenal gland that serves as raw material for the body to make sex hormones; also known as dehydroepiandrosterone
DNA	The molecule that contains the codes for making genes.

Endocrine system	The network of glands and organs in the body that secrete hormones to control and coordinate your body's metabolism, energy level, reproduction, growth and development, mood, and response to injury and stress
Endometriosis	A disease in which tissue similar to the lining of the uterus is found outside the uterus. Endometriosis causes pain and reduces fertility. It is caused by a high level of estradiol compared to progesterone
Endothelium	Single-cell layer of tissue lining the inner walls of blood vessels
Eosinophils	Disease-fighting white blood cells that are activated by food allergies
Estradiol	A hormone that is responsible for a woman's menstrual cycle
Fibrinogen	A protein that causes blood to clot
Free radicals	An unstable form of the oxygen molecule; it carries an electric charge, which allows it to bond with and change cell structures, thereby damaging body tissues and mitochondria
Fructose	A type of sugar from fruits
FSH	Hormone that stimulates the ovaries to secrete progesterone; also known as follicle-stimulating hormone
GH	An inactive hormone secretes during the mature period to determinate the height; also known as growth hormone
Glutathione	An enzyme that neutralizes free radicals
Glycation	The process of joining a molecule of sugar to a protein or fat
HbA1C test	A blood test that shows how much glucose is connected to hemoglobin; also known as hemoglobin A1C test
HDL	The good cholesterol; also known as high-density lipoprotein
Homocysteine	An amino acid that can have an adverse effect on heart health
Hypophysis	gland that is connected to the hypothalamus; also known as the pituitary gland
Hypothalamus	A region located in the lower part of the brain that is connected with every area of the brain. It manages everything that happens in the body and how it reacts to its environment. Also known as the "small brain"
Hippocampus	The memory center of the brain; it stores all the information it receives from the outside or from the body itself.

IGF-1	Active form of the growth hormone; also known as insulin-like growth factor-1
Insulin	Hormone responsible for the utilization of glucose in the body
LDL	The "bad" cholesterol; also known as low-density lipoprotein
LH	The hormone that activates the ovaries to create estradiol; also known as luteinizing hormone
Lymph node	One of many small glands scattered throughout the body that produce white cells and lymphocytes
Melatonin	The sleep hormone; secreted in the pineal gland
Myoma	a benign tumor in the uterus
NAC	N-acetyl cysteine; an antioxidant that increases glutathione and SOD enzymes to neutralize free radicals quickly to prevent tissue and mitochondrial damage
NAD +	A molecule that produces energy in the mitochondria; also known as nicotinamide adenine dinucleotide
Osteopenia	Loss of bone mineral density
Osteoporosis	Severe bone mineral loss
Orexin	An enzyme that is secreted in the brain to maintain alertness and normal weight
Oxytocin	Hormone that contracts the uterus during childbirth and facilitates milk flow for breastfeeding; also known as the "love hormone"
Pancreas	Gland located in the left abdominal area that produces insulin
Papilloma virus	A virus that causes cancer in the uterine cervix
PARP enzymes	A group of enzymes that are active at night and repair damaged DNA, thereby preventing cancer; also known as poly(ADP-ribose) polymerase enzymes
Phytoestrogen	A plant-derived xenoestrogen (see below) with functions similar to those of the hormone estradiol
Prednisone	Steroid drug (non-biological) that reduces inflammation on an autoimmune background
Pregnenolone	Hormone produced by the adrenal glands to improve memory
Progesterone	Hormone that regulates the menstrual cycle and helps convert T4 into T3 in men and women

Prolactin hormone	Hormone that helps produces breast milk after childbirth
PTH	Hormone secreted by the parathyroid gland to help maintain a normal calcium/magnesium balance in the body; also known as parathyroid hormone
PUFAs	Polyunsaturated fatty acids; used to make margarine and animal feed; also used widely in the food industry
Resveratrol	A supplement that works against free radicals and may prevent cancer
rT3	An inactive hormone produced during the conversion of T4 to T3 as a result of dysfunctional 5D activity
SOD	Enzyme that immediately neutralizes free radicals; also known as superoxide dismutase
Statin drugs	Drugs prescribed to lower blood cholesterol
T3	Active thyroid hormone; also known as triiodothyronine
T4	Inactive thyroid hormone or pre-hormone; also known as thyroxine
Thymus gland	A small gland located in the upper chest that is responsible for activating the immune system
TRH	Hormone produced in the hypothalamus to stimulate the pituitary gland to secrete TSH; also known as thyroid-releasing hormone
Triglyceride	The main constituent of fats in the body
TSH	Hormone secreted by the pituitary gland to stimulate the thyroid gland to secrete its hormones; also known as thyroid-stimulating hormone
Vitamin A	A vitamin that is necessary for the secretion of hormones in the thyroid gland
Vitamin C	An antioxidant vitamin
Vitamin D	A vitamin that functions as a hormone to promote bone health and immune system activity
Vitamin E	An antioxidant vitamin
Xenoestrogen	A synthetic industrial chemical that triggers the same pathways as estradiol

Bibliography

Introduction
1. Morley L. van der Berg. Endocrinology of Aging. Humana Press 2000
2. Hertoghe T. The Hormonal Solution. 2002
3. Chand M. Mitochondrial Dysfunction. Kindle Edition
4. Cranton E. Resetting the Clock. 1996
5. James DS. Textbook of Functional Medicine. 2005
6. Klatz R, Goldman R. Anti-Aging Therapies. 1997

Chapter 1: The Mitochondria: The Spring of Life
1. https://www.youtube.com/watch?v=39HTpUG1MwQ
2. https://www.goodreads.com/en/book/show/39793692-the-selfhacked-secrets/page9.
3. Wrutniak-Cabello C, et al. Thyroid hormone action in mitochondria. https://pubmed.ncbi.nlm.nih.gov/11174855/T3
4. Sádaba MC, et al. Insulin-like growth factor 1 (IGF-1) therapy: mitochondrial dysfunction and diseases. https://pubmed.ncbi.nlm.nih.gov/27020404/
5. Vasconsuelo A, et al. Actions of 17-estradiol and testosterone in the mitochondria and their implications in aging. https://pubmed.ncbi.nlm.nih.gov/24041489/
6. Lai C-H, et al. Exercise training enhanced SIRT1 longevity signaling replaces the IGF1 survival pathway to attenuate aging-induced rat heart apoptosis. https://www.ncbi.nlm.nih.gov/pmc/articles/PMC4453937/
7. Cantó C, et al. The NAD+ precursor nicotinamide riboside enhances oxidative metabolism and protects against high-fat diet-induced obesity: cell metabolism. https://pubmed.ncbi.nlm.nih.gov/22682224/
8. Smoliga JM, et al. Resveratrol and health: a comprehensive review of human clinical trials. https://pubmed.ncbi.nlm.nih.gov/21688389/
9. Caton PW. Fructose induces gluconeogenesis and lipogenesis through a SIRT1-depending mechanism. https://joe.bioscientifica.com/view/journals/joe/208/3/273.xml
10. Kramer P, et al. Our (mother's) mitochondria and our mind. https://pubmed.ncbi.nlm.nih.gov/28937858/
11. Garcia-Ruiz C, et al. Mitochondrial glutathione: hepatocellular survival-death switch. https://pubmed.ncbi.nlm.nih.gov/16958667/
12. Nogueiras R, et al. Sirtuin 1 and Sirtuin 3: physiological modulators of metabolism. https://www.ncbi.nlm.nih.gov/pmc/articles/PMC3746174/
13. Shin-ichiro Imai ,et al. NAD+ and sirtuins in aging and disease. https://pubmed.ncbi.nlm.nih.gov/24786309/NAD

14. Cohen J. Understand why you're sick and how to get well. https://www.goodreads.com/en/book/show/39793692-the-selfhacked-secrets/ page 46.
15. Zink AN, et al. The orexin neuropeptide system: physical activity and hypothalamic function throughout the aging process. https://www.ncbi.nlm.nih.gov/pmc/articles/PMC4219460/
16. Pascal JM. The comings and goings of PARP-1 in response to DNA damage. https://pubmed.ncbi.nlm.nih.gov/30177435/16.
17. Dantzer F., et al. Poly(ADP-ribose) polymerase-1 activation during DNA damage and repair. https://pubmed.ncbi.nlm.nih.gov/16793420
18. Rovira-Llopis S, et al. Mitochondrial dynamics in type 2 diabetes: pathophysiological implications. https://pubmed.ncbi.nlm.nih.gov/28131082/
19. Ames BN. Low micronutrient intake may accelerate the degenerative diseases of aging through allocation of scarce micronutrients by triage. https://www.ncbi.nlm.nih.gov/pmc/articles/PMC1693790/
20. Chow J, et al. Mitochondrial disease and endocrine dysfunction. https://pubmed.ncbi.nlm.nih.gov/27716753/
21. Cristen CG, et al. Chronically alternating light cycles increase breast cancer risk in mice: Current Biology (cell.com). https://www.ncbi.nlm.nih.gov/pmc/articles/PMC1693790/

Chapter 2: My personal experience with natural hormone therapy

1. Parker DC, Judd HL, et al. Pubertal sleep-wake patterns of episodic LH, FSH and testosterone release in twin boys. Pubmed.ncbi.nlm.nih.gov/1169258/
2. Gardner K. https://www.livestrong.com/article/320492-the-effects-of-eating-late-at-night/
3. Iranmanesh A, Lawson D, Johannes D. Glucose ingestion acutely lowers pulsatile LH and basal testosterone secretion in men. https://pubmed.ncbi.nlm.nih.gov/22252939/
4. Berryman DE, et al. The GH/IGF-1 axis in obesity: pathophysiology and therapeutic considerations. https://www.nature.com/articles/nrendo.2013.64
5. Reineh T. Obesity and thyroid function. https://pubmed.ncbi.nlm.nih.gov/19540303.
6. Kraemer WJ, et al. Recovery responses of testosterone, growth hormone, and IGF-1 after resistance exercise. https://pubmed.ncbi.nlm.nih.gov/27856715
7. Iranmanesh A, et al. Glucose ingestion acutely lowers pulsatile LH and basal testosterone secretion in men. https://pubmed.ncbi.nlm.nih.gov/22252939/
8. Jensen TK, et al. Habitual alcohol consumption associated with reduced semen quality and changes in reproductive hormones; a cross-sectional

study among 1221 young Danish men. https://pubmed.ncbi.nlm.nih.gov/25277121/

9. Rudman D, et al. Effects of human growth hormone in men over 60 years old. https://pubmed.ncbi.nlm.nih.gov/2355952/

10. Masters A, et al. Melatonin, the hormone of darkness: from sleep promotion to Ebola treatment. https://pubmed.ncbi.nlm.nih.gov/25705578/

11. Labrie F. DHEA: important source of sex steroids in men and even more in women. https://pubmed.ncbi.nlm.nih.gov/20541662/

12. Osuji IJ, et al. Pregnenolone for cognition and mood in dual diagnosis patients. https://pubmed.ncbi.nlm.nih.gov/20493557/

13. Strous RD, et al. Analysis of neurosteroid levels in attention deficit hyperactivity disorder. https://academic.oup.com/ijnp/article/4/3/259/976221

14. Ferrari E, et al. Age-related changes of the hypothalamic-pituitary-adrenal axis: pathophysiological correlates. https://pubmed.ncbi.nlm.nih.gov/11275940/HPA

15. Gardner K. Carbs before bed. https://www.livestrong.com/article/320492-the-effects-of-eating-late-at-night/

16. Hunter H. We are what we eat: the link between diet, evolution and non-genetic inheritance. https://www.ncbi.nlm.nih.gov/pmc/articles/PMC2373379/

17. Tabachnick M, et al. Effect of long-chain fatty acids on the binding of thyroxine and triiodothyronine to human thyroxine-binding globulin. http://www.ncbi.nlm.nih.gov/pubmed/2869786

18. Fukusen N, et al. Inhibition of chymase activity by phosphoglycerides. https://pubmed.ncbi.nlm.nih.gov/3882053/

19. Tabachnick M, et al. Effect of long-chain fatty acids on the binding of thyroxine and triiodothyronine to human thyroxine-binding globulin. http://www.ncbi.nlm.nih.gov/pubmed/2869786

20. Chopra IJ, et al. Evidence for an inhibitor of extrathyroidal conversion of thyroxine to 3,5,3' triiodothyronine in sera of patients with nonthyroidal illnesses. http://www.ncbi.nlm.nih.gov/pubmed/2857729

21. Wiersinga WM, et al. Inhibition of nuclear T3 binding by fatty acids. http://www.ncbi.nlm.ni.gov/pubmed/3173114.

22. Rafael J, et al. The effect of essential fatty acid deficiency on basal respiration and function of liver mitochondria in rats. http://www.ncbi.nlm.nih.gov/pubmed/6693988

23. Hu M, et al. Polyunsaturated fatty acid intake and incidence of type 2 diabetes in adults: a dose response meta-analysis of cohort studies. https://dmsjournal.biomedcentral.com/articles/10.1186/s13098-022-00804-1

24. Xiaoxi Li et al., Therapeutic potential of []-3 polyunsaturated fatty acids in human autoimmune diseases. https://www.ncbi.nlm.nih.gov/pmc/articles/PMC6776881/

Chapter 3: The huge biological role of the thyroid gland

1. de Vries EM et al. The molecular basis of the non-thyroidal illness syndrome. https://pubmed.ncbi.nlm.nih.gov/25972358/
2. Jonklaas J et al. Guidelines for the Treatment of Hypothyroidism: Prepared by the American Thyroid Association Task Force on Thyroid Hormone Replacement. https://www.ncbi.nlm.nih.gov/pmc/articles/PMC4267409/.
3. Gomes-Lima C, et al. Can reverse T3 assay be employed to guide T4 vs T4/T3 therapy in hypothyroidism? https://www.frontiersin.org/articles/10.3389/fendo.2019.00856/full
4. Mancini A, et al. Thyroid hormones, oxidative stress, and inflammation. https://pubmed.ncbi.nlm.nih.gov/27051079/
5. Liontiris MI, et al. A concise review of Hashimoto thyroiditis (HT) and the importance of iodine, selenium, vitamin D and gluten on the autoimmunity and dietary management of HT patients. Points that need more investigation. https://pubmed.ncbi.nlm.nih.gov/28315909/
6. Ambooken B, et al. Zinc deficiency associated with hypothyroidism: an overlooked cause of severe alopecia https://pubmed.ncbi.nlm.nih.gov/23960398/
7. Schroffner WG. The aging thyroid in health and disease. https://pubmed.ncbi.nlm.nih.gov/3110016/
8. Wallace K, et al. Thyroid dysfunction: how to manage overt and subclinical disease in older patients. https://pubmed.ncbi.nlm.nih.gov/9559026/
9. Crawford M, et al. Testosterone replacement therapy: role of pituitary and thyroid in diagnosis and treatment. https://pubmed.ncbi.nlm.nih.gov/28078216/
10. Akande EO. Plasma concentration of gonadotrophins, oestrogen and progesterone in hypothyroid women. https://pubmed.ncbi.nlm.nih.gov/1148139/
11. Khanderia U, et al. Amiodarone-induced thyroid dysfunction. https://pubmed.ncbi.nlm.nih.gov/8258259/
12. Batcheret EL, al. Thyroid function abnormalities during amiodarone therapy for persistent atrial fibrillation. https://pubmed.ncbi.nlm.nih.gov/17904459/
13. Heyma P et al. Glucocorticoids decrease in conversion of thyroxine into 3, 5, 3'-tri-iodothyronine by isolated rat renal tubules. https://pubmed.ncbi.nlm.nih.gov/7053919/
14. Torino F, et al. Thyroid dysfunction as an unintended side effect of anti-cancer drugs. https://pubmed.ncbi.nlm.nih.gov/23750887/
15. Heyma P, et al. D-propranolol and L-propranolol both decrease conversion of L-thyroxine to L-triiodothyronine. https://pubmed.ncbi.nlm.nih.gov/7407482/

16. Sorger D, et al. Effects of various contraceptives on laboratory parameters in diagnosis of thyroid gland function with special reference to the free hormones FT4 and FT3. https://pubmed.ncbi.nlm.nih.gov/1585690/

17. Berta E, et al. Effect of thyroid hormone status and concomitant medication on statin induced adverse effects in hyperlipidemic patients. https://pubmed.ncbi.nlm.nih.gov/24974574/

18. Coyle PV, et al. Epstein-Barr virus infection and thyroid dysfunction. https://pubmed.ncbi.nlm.nih.gov/2564972/

19. Parsa AA, et al. HIV and thyroid dysfunction. https://pubmed.ncbi.nlm.nih.gov/23743889/

20. Ho HC, et al. Hypothyroidism and adrenal insufficiency in sepsis and hemorrhagic shock. https://pubmed.ncbi.nlm.nih.gov/15545567/

21. Cerillo AG. The low triiodothyronine syndrome: a strong predictor of low cardiac output and death in patients undergoing coronary artery bypass grafting. https://pubmed.ncbi.nlm.nih.gov/24636708/

22. Worku B. Preoperative hypothyroidism is a risk factor for postoperative atrial fibrillation in cardiac surgical patients. https://pubmed.ncbi.nlm.nih.gov/25640607/

23. Fauci AS, Braunwald E, Kasper DC, et al. Harrison's Principles of Internal Medicine, 17th edition. New York: McGraw-Hill Professional; 2008.

24. Lado-Abeal J. Thyroid hormones are needed to sustain "inappropriately" normal TSH during non-thyroidal illness syndrome: a clinical observation in severely ill patients with primary hypothyroidism. https://pubmed.ncbi.nlm.nih.gov/25789598/

25. Wilson. Low body temperature with normal thyroid blood test. https://www.wilsonssyndrome.com/identify/wts-overview/

26. Burroughs V, et al. Thyroid function in the elderly. https://pubmed.ncbi.nlm.nih.gov/6798870/

27. Kilic M, et al. The effect of exhaustion exercise on thyroid hormones and testosterone levels of elite athletes receiving oral zinc. http://www.ncbi.nlm.nih.gov/pubmed/16648789

28. Faigin R. Natural Hormonal Enhancement. Extique (internet publisher); 2000: page 265.

29. Agha-Hosseini F, et al. The association of elevated plasma cortisol and Hashimoto's Thyroiditis, a neglected part of immune response. https://pubmed.ncbi.nlm.nih.gov/27075805/

30. Evelyn L Jara et al. Modulating the function of the immune system by thyroid hormones and thyrotropin. https://pubmed.ncbi.nlm.nih.gov/28216261/

31. Lee J. Human body temperature has decreased in United States, study finds. https://med.stanford.edu/news/all-news/2020/01/human-body-temperature-has-decreased-in-united-states.html.

32. Habersaat KB, et al. Pandemic fatigue: reinvigorating the public to prevent COVID-19. Policy framework for supporting pandemic prevention and management https://reliefweb.int/report/world/pandemic-fatigue-reinvigorating-public-prevent-covid-19-policy-framework-supporting?gclid=CjOKCQiAz9ieBhCIARIsACBOoGK15zP1Um_NML206WRucSbCjhvSanj9FKZziXBjqP1QDwJp0e3ir4UaAilIEALw_wcB WHO

33. Iacovides S, et al. Could the ketogenic diet induce a shift in thyroid function and support a metabolic advantage in healthy participants? A pilot randomized-controlled-crossover trial. https://pubmed.ncbi.nlm.nih.gov/35658056/ketogenic diet affect thyroid function

34. Farhangi MA, et al The effect of vitamin A supplementation on thyroid function in premenopausal women. https://pubmed.ncbi.nlm.nih.gov/23378454/

35. Lies, Damned Lies, and Statistics. https://www.highpoint-associates.com/2017/06/lies-damned-lies-statistics/

Chapter 4: The mystery disease called hypothyroidism

- Bowthorpe J at al. Stop the thyroid madness II. 2014.
- Fogel WA. Diamine oxidase (DAO) and female sex hormones. https://pubmed.ncbi.nlm.nih.gov/3088928/
- Udovcic MA, et al. Hypothyroidism and the Heart. https://www.ncbi.nlm.nih.gov/pmc/articles/PMC5512679/
- Dittfeld A, et al. A possible link between the Epstein-Barr virus infection and autoimmune thyroid disorders. https://www.ncbi.nlm.nih.gov/pmc/articles/PMC5099387/
- Basile LM, et al. COVID-19 and post-infection thyroid disease. https://www.endocrineweb.com/covid-19-post-infection-thyroid-disease
- Bunevicius, R, et al. Effects of thyroxine as compared with thyroxine plus triiodothyronine in patients with hypothyroidism. https://pubmed.ncbi.nlm.nih.gov/9971866/
- Kaliaperuma R, et al. Relationship between lipoprotein(a) and thyroid hormones in hypothyroid patients. https://pubmed.ncbi.nlm.nih.gov/24701476/
- Cerillo AG. The low triiodothyronine syndrome: a strong predictor of low cardiac output and death in patients undergoing coronary artery bypass grafting. https://pubmed.ncbi.nlm.nih.gov/24636708/
- Verhoef P, et al. Contribution of caffeine to the homocysteine-raising effect of coffee: a randomized controlled trial in humans. https://pubmed.ncbi.nlm.nih.gov/12450889/
- Abu-Taha M, et al. Combined effect of coffee consumption and cigarette smoking on serum levels of vitamin B12, folic acid, and lipid profile in

young male: a cross-sectional study. https://www.ncbi.nlm.nih.gov/pmc/articles/PMC6878925/

- Gilfix BM. Vitamin B12 and homocysteine. https://www.ncbi.nlm.nih.gov/pmc/articles/PMC1283514/
- Delitala PA. et al. Thyroid hormone diseases and osteoporosis. https://pubmed.ncbi.nlm.nih.gov/32268542/
- Shafran S.D. The chronic fatigue syndrome. https://www.sciencedirect.com/science/article/abs/pii/S0002934305800634.
- Protsiv M. Ley C. Lankester J. Hastie T. Parsonnet. J. Decreasing human body temperature in the United States since the Industrial Revolution. https://elifesciences.org/articles/49555

Chapter 5: Your complaints due to the lack of T3 in tissues

1. Bowthorpe J, et al. Stop the thyroid madness II. 2014.
2. Fogel WA. Diamine oxidase (DAO) and female sex hormones. https://pubmed.ncbi.nlm.nih.gov/3088928/
3. Maja Udovci et al. Hypothyroidism and the heart. https://www.ncbi.nlm.nih.gov/pmc/articles/PMC5512679/
4. Cortés C, et al. Hypothyroidism in the adult rat causes incremental changes in brain-derived neurotrophic factor, neuronal and astrocyte apoptosis, gliosis, and deterioration of postsynaptic density. https://www.ncbi.nlm.nih.gov/pmc/articles/PMC3429274/
5. Dittfeld A, et al. A possible link between the Epstein-Barr virus infection and autoimmune thyroid disorders. https://www.ncbi.nlm.nih.gov/pmc/articles/PMC5099387/
6. Rudroff T, et al. Post-COVID-19 fatigue: potential contributing factors. https://pubmed.ncbi.nlm.nih.gov/33352638/
7. Townsend L, et al. Persistent fatigue following SARS-CoV-2 infection is common and independent of severity of initial infection. https://pubmed.ncbi.nlm.nih.gov/33166287/
8. Aliaperumal R, et al. Relationship between lipoprotein(a) and thyroid hormones in hypothyroid patients. https://pubmed.ncbi.nlm.nih.gov/24701476/
9. Cerillo AG, et al. The low triiodothyronine syndrome: a strong predictor of low cardiac output and death in patients undergoing coronary artery bypass grafting. https://pubmed.ncbi.nlm.nih.gov/24636708/
10. Verhoef P, et al. Contribution of caffeine to the homocysteine-raising effect of coffee: a randomized controlled trial in humans. https://pubmed.ncbi.nlm.nih.gov/12450889/
11. Abu-Taha, M et al. Combined effect of coffee consumption and cigarette smoking on serum levels of vitamin B12, folic acid, and lipid profile in

young male: a cross-sectional study. https://www.ncbi.nlm.nih.gov/pmc/articles/PMC6878925/

12. Varga EA, et al. Homocysteine and MTHFR mutations. Relation to thrombosis and coronary artery disease. https://www.ahajournals.org/doi/full/10.1161/01.CIR.0000165142.37711.E7.

13. Gilfix BM. Vitamin B12 and homocysteine. https://www.ncbi.nlm.nih.gov/pmc/articles/PMC1283514/

14. Gillberg IC. Hypothyroidism and autism spectrum disorders https://pubmed.ncbi.nlm.nih.gov/1577897/

15. Delitala AP, et al. Thyroid hormone diseases and osteoporosis. https://pubmed.ncbi.nlm.nih.gov/32268542/

16. Smith TS. Cancer scientists point finger at T4 & RT3 hormones. https://thyroidpatients.ca/2020/02/05/cancer-scientists-point-finger-at-t4-rt3-hormones/.

17. Wang SH, et al. 2-Methoxyestradiol, an endogenous estrogen metabolite, induces thyroid cell apoptosis. https://pubmed.ncbi.nlm.nih.gov/10940494/

18. Muneyyirci-Delale O, et al. Serum ionized magnesium and calcium in women after men. https://www.ncbi.nlm.nih.gov/pubmed/10231048

19. Heyma P. Glucocorticoids decrease the conversion of thyroxine into 3,5,3'-tri-iodothyronine by isolated rat renal tubules. http://www.clinsci.org/content/62/2/215

20. Shoemaker C. Chronic stress and hypothyroidism. https://sanescohealth.com/blog/chronic-stress-hypothyroidism/

21. Ocklenburg S. The serotonin transporter gene and depression. https://www.psychologytoday.com/us/blog/the-asymmetric-brain/201905/

22. Touma TB, et al. Liothyronine for depression: a review and guidance for safety monitoring. https://www.ncbi.nlm.nih.gov/pmc/articles/PMC5451035/

23. Morin AK. Triiodothyronine (T3) supplementation in major depressive disorder. https://meridian.allenpress.com/mhc/article/5/6/253/127788/Triiodothyronine-T3-supplementation-in-major

24. Rosen A. How stress affects child development. https://centerforanxietydisorders.com/stress-affects-child-development/

25. Rone J K, et al. The effect of endurance training on serum triiodothyronine kinetics in man: physical conditioning marked by enhanced thyroid hormone metabolism. https://pubmed.ncbi.nlm.nih.gov/1483287/

26. Scott E. Cortisol is a naturally occurring steroid known as the stress hormone.https://www.verywellmind.com/cortisol-and-depression-1066764

27. Young SN. How to increase serotonin in the human brain without drugs. https://www.ncbi.nlm.nih.gov/pmc/articles/PMC2077351/

28. Knechtle B, et al. Physiology and pathophysiology in ultra-marathon running. https://pubmed.ncbi.nlm.nih.gov/29910741/
29. Tafet GE, et al. Correlation between cortisol level and serotonin uptake in patients with chronic stress and depression. https://pubmed.ncbi.nlm.nih.gov/12467090/
30. Zhang Y, et al. Prolactin and thyroid stimulating hormone (TSH) levels and sexual dysfunction in patients with schizophrenia treated with conventional antipsychotic medication: a cross-sectional study. https://pubmed.ncbi.nlm.nih.gov/30554232/
31. Shimoyama N, et al. Serum thyroid hormone levels correlate with cardiac function and ventricular tachyarrhythmia in patients with chronic heart failure. https://europepmc.org/article/med/8176632
32. Rawla P, et al. IgA deficiency. https://www.ncbi.nlm.nih.gov/books/NBK538205/
33. García-Ruiz C et al. Mitochondrial cholesterol in health and disease. https://pubmed.ncbi.nlm.nih.gov/19012251/
34. Rui L. Energy metabolism in the liver. https://pubmed.ncbi.nlm.nih.gov/24692138/
35. C. Canto et al. The NAD+ precursor nicotidine ribose enhances oxidative metabolism and protects against high fat diet-induced obesity. https://www.cell.com/cell-metabolism/fulltext/S1550-4131(12)00192-1
36. García-Ruiz C et al. Mitochondrial cholesterol and the paradox in cell death. https://pubmed.ncbi.nlm.nih.gov/28035533/
37. Siri-Torino PW et al. Saturated fatty acids and risk of coronary heart disease: modulation by replacement nutrients. https://www.ncbi.nlm.nih.gov/pmc/articles/PMC2943062/
38. Bowden J, Sinatra S. The Great Cholesterol Myth: Why Lowering Your Cholesterol Won't Prevent Heart Disease and the Statin-Free Plan That Will. Beverly, MA: Fair Winds Press; 2012.

Are high blood glucose levels related to thyroid gland activity?

1. Rovira-Llopis S, et al. Mitochondrial dynamics in type 2 diabetes: pathophysiological implications. https://pubmed.ncbi.nlm.nih.gov/28131082/
2. Pinti M. V et al. Mitochondrial dysfunction in type 2 diabetes mellitus: an organ-based analysis. https://pubmed.ncbi.nlm.nih.gov/30601700/Type

Is obesity related to thyroid gland activity?

1. Iranmanesh A, et al. Glucose ingestion acutely lowers pulsatile LH and basal testosterone secretion in men. Am J Physiol Endocrinol Metab. 2012;302(6):30-E724.
2. Afaghi A et al. High-glycemic-index carbohydrate meals shorten sleep onset. Am J Clin Nutr. 2007;85(2):30-426.

3. Chandler-Laney PC, et al. Return of hunger following a relatively high carbohydrate breakfast is associated with earlier recorded glucose peak and nadir. https://www.ncbi.nlm.nih.gov/pmc/articles/PMC4204795/
4. Gibbon CH, et al. Experimental hypoglycemia is a human model of stress-induced hyperalgesia. https://pubmed.ncbi.nlm.nih.gov/22921261/
5. Pernet A, et al. Transient triiodothyronine deficiency: absence of effect on basal or adrenaline-stimulated carbohydrate and lipid metabolism in man. https://pubmed.ncbi.nlm.nih.gov/7047251/
6. Scott KP et al. The influence of diet on the gut microbiota. https://pubmed.ncbi.nlm.nih.gov/23147033/
7. Odenwald MA, et al. Intestinal permeability defects: is it time to treat? https://pubmed.ncbi.nlm.nih.gov/23851019/
8. Farshchi MK, et al. A viewpoint on the leaky gut syndrome to treat allergic asthma: a novel opinion. https://pubmed.ncbi.nlm.nih.gov/30208732/

Is coronary artery disease related to thyroid gland hypoactivity?

1. von Hafe M, et al. The impact of thyroid hormone dysfunction on ischemic heart disease. https://pubmed.ncbi.nlm.nih.gov/30959486/
2. Biondi B, et al. Subclinical hypothyroidism and cardiac function. https://pubmed.ncbi.nlm.nih.gov/12165114/
3. Jabbar A, et al. Thyroid hormones and cardiovascular disease. https://pubmed.ncbi.nlm.nih.gov/27811932/
4. Ertugrul O, et al. Prevalence of subclinical hypothyroidism among patients with acute myocardial infarction. https://www.hindawi.com/journals/isrn/2011/810251/

Chapter 6: Cases Reported

1. F.Keen at al.Anti-psychotic drugs and thyroid function. https://etj.bioscientifica.com/view/journals/etj/11/2/ETJ-21-0119.xml central hypothyroidism related to antipsychotic drugs.
2. Bunevicius R, Steibliene V, Prange AJ. Thyroid axis function after in-patient treatment of acute psychosis with antipsychotics: a naturalistic study. BMC Psychiatry. 2014; 14(279). doi:10.1186/s12888-014-0279-7
3. Faiging RJD. Natural Hormonal Enhancement. (Internet) Extique; 2000.
4. Lai E CC, Yang Y-H K, Lin S-J, Hsieh C-Y. Use of anti-epileptic drugs and risk of hypothyroidism. https://pubmed.ncbi.nlm.nih.gov/23946049/
5. Yilmaz U, Yilmaz TS, Akinci G, Korkmaz HA, Tekgul H. The effect of anti-epileptic drugs on thyroid function in children. https://pubmed.ncbi.nlm.nih.gov/24091037/ITEM.
6. Zhang Y, Tang Z, Ruan Y, et al. Prolactin and thyroid stimulating hormone (TSH) levels and sexual dysfunction in patients with schizophrenia treated with conventional antipsychotic medication: a cross-sectional study. https://pubmed.ncbi.nlm.nih.gov/30554232/

Chapter 7: Thyroid Gland and Immune Diseases

1. Chen-Yen Yang, et al. The implication of vitamin D and autoimmunity: a comprehensive review. https://www.ncbi.nlm.nih.gov/pmc/articles/PMC6047889/
2. Barbara Altieri, et al. Does vitamin D play a role in autoimmune endocrine disorders? A proof of concept. https://pubmed.ncbi.nlm.nih.gov/28070798/
3. Mora JR, et al. Vitamin effects on the immune system: vitamins A and D take center stage. https://pubmed.ncbi.nlm.nih.gov/19172691/
4. Obrenovich MEM. Leaky gut, leaky brain. https://pubmed.ncbi.nlm.nih.gov/30340384/?
5. Lerner A, et al. Adverse effects of gluten ingestion and advantages of gluten withdrawal in nonceliac autoimmune disease. https://pubmed.ncbi.nlm.nih.gov/29202198/
6. Shmerling RH. Autoimmune disease and stress: Is there a link? https://www.health.harvard.edu/blog/autoimmune-disease-and-stress-is-there-a-link-2018071114230
7. Salter DR, et at. Triiodothyronine (T3) and cardiovascular therapeutics: a review. https://pubmed.ncbi.nlm.nih.gov/1482831/
8. Nederstigt C, et al. Associated auto-immune disease in type 1 diabetes patients: a systematic review and meta-analysis https://pubmed.ncbi.nlm.nih.gov/30508413/
9. Rayman MP. Multiple nutritional factors and thyroid disease, with particular reference to autoimmune thyroid disease https://pubmed.ncbi.nlm.nih.gov/30208979/
10. Faber J, Cohn D, et al. Subclinical hypothyroidism in Addison's disease. https://pubmed.ncbi.nlm.nih.gov/494979//
11. Pompella A, et al. The changing faces of glutathione, a cellular protagonist https://pubmed.ncbi.nlm.nih.gov/14555227/
12. Wang SH, et al. 2-Methoxyestradiol, an endogenous estrogen metabolite, induces thyroid cell apoptosis https://pubmed.ncbi.nlm.nih.gov/10940494/
13. Wiersinga WM. T4 + T3 combination therapy: any progress? https://pubmed.ncbi.nlm.nih.gov/31617166/
14. Abhik R, et al. Prevalence of celiac disease in patients with autoimmune thyroid disease: a meta-analysis https://pubmed.ncbi.nlm.nih.gov/27256300/
15. Souto Filho JT, et al. Predictive risk factors for autoimmune thyroid diseases in patients with pernicious anemia. https://pubmed.ncbi.nlm.nih.gov/31780218/?
16. Freeman HAJ. Endocrine manifestations in celiac disease. https://pubmed.ncbi.nlm.nih.gov/27784959/

17. Baldini C, et al. The Association of Sjögren Syndrome and Autoimmune Thyroid Disorders https://www.ncbi.nlm.nih.gov/pmc/articles/PMC5891591/
18. Vicente Robazz TCM, et al. Autoimmune thyroid disease in patients with rheumatic diseases. https://pubmed.ncbi.nlm.nih.gov/22641595/
19. Luo W, et al. Association between systemic lupus erythematosus and thyroid dysfunction: a meta-analysis https://pubmed.ncbi.nlm.nih.gov/30376437/
20. Antonelli A, et al. Fatigue in patients with systemic sclerosis and hypothyroidism: a review of the literature and report of our experience. https://pubmed.ncbi.nlm.nih.gov/28375832/multiple sclerosis
21. D'Intino G, et al. Triiodothyronine administration ameliorates the demyelination/remyelination ratio in a non-human primate model of multiple sclerosis by correcting tissue hypothyroidism. https://pubmed.ncbi.nlm.nih.gov/21707794/
22. Ruiz-Núñez B. Higher prevalence of "low T3 syndrome" in patients with chronic fatigue syndrome: a case-control study. https://pubmed.ncbi.nlm.nih.gov/29615976/
23. Fazzi P, et al. Sarcoidosis and thyroid autoimmunity. https://pubmed.ncbi.nlm.nih.gov/28848497/
24. Fliers E. Thyroid function in critically ill patients. https://pubmed.ncbi.nlm.nih.gov/26071885/

Chapter 8: Disorders in the women menstrual cycle

1. Heyma P, et al. Glucocorticoids decrease in conversion of thyroxine into 3, 5, 3'-tri-iodothyronine by isolated rat renal tubules. https://pubmed.ncbi.nlm.nih.gov/7053919/
2. Sathyapalan T, et al. The effect of soy phytoestrogen supplementation on thyroid status and cardiovascular risk markers in patients with subclinical hypothyroidism: a randomized, double-blind, crossover study. https://pubmed.ncbi.nlm.nih.gov/21325465/
3. Montes-Grajales, et al. Computer-aided identification of novel protein targets of bisphenol A. https://pubmed.ncbi.nlm.nih.gov/23973438/
4. Mancini. Thyroid hormones, oxidative stress, and inflammation. https://pubmed.ncbi.nlm.nih.gov/27051079/
5. Subbaramaiah K, et al. Obesity is associated with inflammation and elevated aromatase expression in the mouse mammary gland. https://pubmed.ncbi.nlm.nih.gov/21372033/
6. Hertel J, et al. Evidence for stress-like alterations in the HPA-axis in women taking oral contraceptives. https://pubmed.ncbi.nlm.nih.gov/29074884/ oral contraceptives

7. Skovlund CW, et al. Association of hormonal contraception with depression. https://pubmed.ncbi.nlm.nih.gov/27680324/

8. Mørch LS, et al. Contemporary hormonal contraception and the risk of breast cancer. https://pubmed.ncbi.nlm.nih.gov/29211679/

9. Cauci S, et al. Combined oral contraceptives increase high-sensitivity c-reactive protein but not haptoglobin in female athletes. https://pubmed.ncbi.nlm.nih.gov/27084393/

10. Khalili H, et al. Oral contraceptives, reproductive factors and risk of inflammatory bowel disease. https://pubmed.ncbi.nlm.nih.gov/22619368/

11. Kowalska KA, et al. Pro/antioxidant status in young healthy women using oral contraceptives. https://pubmed.ncbi.nlm.nih.gov/26921793/

12. Moloney JN, et al. ROS signaling in the biology of cancer. https://pubmed.ncbi.nlm.nih.gov/28587975/

13. Valko M, et al. Free radicals, metals and antioxidants in oxidative stress-induced cancer. https://pubmed.ncbi.nlm.nih.gov/16430879/

14. Dos Santos CN, et al. Elevation of oxidized lipoprotein of low density in users of combined oral contraceptives. https://pubmed.ncbi.nlm.nih.gov/30328945/

15. Women's Health Initiative Investigators. https://jamanetwork.com/journals/jama/fullarticle/195120

16. Rossouw JE, et al. Risks and benefits of estrogen plus progestin in healthy postmenopausal women: principal results From the Women's Health Initiative randomized controlled trial. https://pubmed.ncbi.nlm.nih.gov/12117397/

17. Gierisch JM, et al. Oral contraceptive use and risk of breast, cervical, colorectal, and endometrial cancers: a systematic review. https://pubmed.ncbi.nlm.nih.gov/24014598/

18. Stephenson K. The effects of compounded bioidentical transdermal hormone therapy on hemostatic, inflammatory, immune factors; cardiovascular biomarkers; quality-of-life measures; and health outcomes in perimenopausal and postmenopausal women. https://pubmed.ncbi.nlm.nih.gov/23627249/ https://pubmed.ncbi.nlm.nih.gov/6513559/ increased estradiol in utero tissues cell.

19. Cavalieri EL, et al. Critical depurinating DNA adducts: estrogen adducts in the etiology and prevention of cancer and dopamine adducts in the etiology and prevention of Parkinson's disease. https://pubmed.ncbi.nlm.nih.gov/28388839/ https://pubmed.ncbi.nlm.nih.gov/28479355/ development of breast cancer.

20. Zhou X. Disturbance of mammary UDP-glucuronosyltransferase represses estrogen metabolism and exacerbates experimental breast cancer. https://www.hindawi.com/journals/isrn/2013/784520/

Chapter 9. Hidden hypothyroidism and pregnancy
1. https://www.hopkinsmedicine.org/health/conditions-and-diseases/staying-healthy-during-pregnancy/hypothyroidism-and-pregnancy.
2. Moog NK, et al. Influence of maternal thyroid hormones during gestation on fetal brain development. https://www.ncbi.nlm.nih.gov/pmc/articles/PMC4819012/
3. Lerner RK, et al. Congenital heart disease and thyroid dysfunction: combination, association, and implication. https://pubmed.ncbi.nlm.nih.gov/31496400/
4. Negro R, et al. Diagnosis and management of subclinical hypothyroidism in pregnancy. https://pubmed.ncbi.nlm.nih.gov/25288580/
5. Gannon AW, et al. https://kidshealth.org/en/parents/congenital-hypothyroidism.html.
6. Nazarpour S, et al. Thyroid dysfunction and pregnancy outcomes. https://pubmed.ncbi.nlm.nih.gov/21212091/
7. Pemberton HN, et al. Thyroid hormones and fetal brain development. https://pubmed.ncbi.nlm.nih.gov/16170282/
8. Blankfield A. Kynurenine pathway pathologies: do nicotinamide and other pathway co-factors have a therapeutic role in reduction of symptom severity, including chronic fatigue syndrome (CFS) and fibromyalgia (FM). https://pubmed.ncbi.nlm.nih.gov/23922501/
9. Al-Nimer MSM, et al. Serum levels of serotonin as a biomarker of newly diagnosed fibromyalgia in women: its relation to the platelet indices. https://www.ncbi.nlm.nih.gov/pmc/articles/PMC6116663/
10. Dukowicz, C, et al. Small intestinal bacterial overgrowth. https://www.ncbi.nlm.nih.gov/pmc/articles/PMC3099351/
11. Iwakur Y, et al. The roles of IL-17A in inflammatory immune responses and host defense against pathogens. https://pubmed.ncbi.nlm.nih.gov/19161416/
12. Chang SH, et al. Vitamin D suppresses Th17 cytokine production by inducing C/EBP homologous protein (CHOP) expression. https://pubmed.ncbi.nlm.nih.gov/20974859/

Chapter 11: Is ADHD in children related to thyroid activity
1. Laake & Compart PJ. https://www.bookdepository.com/The-ADHD-and-Autism-Nutritional-Supplement-Handbook. Attention-Deficit/Hyperactivity Disorder (ADHD). https://www.nimh.nih.gov/health/statistics/attention-deficit-hyperactivity-disorder-adhd
2. Weiss RE, et al. Attention-deficit hyperactivity disorder and thyroid function. https://pubmed.ncbi.nlm.nih.gov/8410504/
3. Gillberg IC, et al. Hypothyroidism and autism spectrum disorders.
4. https://pubmed.ncbi.nlm.nih.gov/1577897/

5. Mengqin Ge, et al. Maternal thyroid dysfunction during pregnancy and the risk of adverse outcomes in the offspring: a systematic review and meta-analysis. https://pubmed.ncbi.nlm.nih.gov/32810262/

6. Rasmussen P, et al. Natural outcome of ADHD with developmental coordination disorder at age 22 years: a controlled, longitudinal, community-based study. http://www.ncbi.nlm.nih.gov/pubmed/11068898

7. Mannuzza S, et al. Long-term prognosis in attention-deficit/hyperactivity disorder. http://www.ncbi.nlm.nih.gov/pubmed/10944664

8. Brookes K-J, et al. A common haplotype of the dopamine transporter gene associated with attention-deficit/hyperactivity disorder and interacting with maternal use of alcohol during pregnancy. http://www.ncbi.nlm.nih.gov/sites/entrez/16389200

9. Thapa, et al. Catechol O-methyltransferase gene variant and birth weight predict early-onset antisocial behavior in children with attention-deficit/hyperactivity disorder. http://www.ncbi.nlm.nih.gov/sites/entrez/16275815

10. Woodruff TJ, et al. Trends in environmentally related childhood illnesses. http://www.ncbi.nlm.nih.gov/sites/entrez/15060210

11. Curtis LT, et al. Nutritional and environmental approaches to preventing and treating autism and attention deficit hyperactivity disorder (ADHD): a review http://www.ncbi.nlm.nih.gov/sites/entrez/18199019

12. Colter L, et al. Fatty acid status and behavioral symptoms of attention deficit hyperactivity disorder in adolescents: a case-control study. http://www.ncbi.nlm.nih.gov/sites/entrez/18275609

13. le Coutre J, et al. Food ingredients and cognitive performance. http://www.ncbi.nlm.nih.gov/pubmed/18827573

14. Zhang X, et al. A high-fat diet rich in saturated and mono-unsaturated fatty acids induces disturbance of thyroid lipid profile and hypothyroxinemia in male rats. https://pubmed.ncbi.nlm.nih.gov/29363248/

15. Ford JD, et al. Child maltreatment, other trauma exposure, and posttraumatic symptomatology among children with oppositional defiant and attention deficit hyperactivity disorders. http://www.ncbi.nlm.nih.gov/sites/entrez/11232267

16. Geller B, et al. Diagnostic characteristics of 93 cases of a prepubertal and early adolescent bipolar disorder phenotype by gender, puberty and comorbid attention deficit hyperactivity disorder. http://www.ncbi.nlm.nih.gov/pubmed/11052405

17. Farrar R, Ferar R, et al. A comparison of the visual symptoms between ADD/ADHD and normal children. https://pubmed.ncbi.nlm.nih.gov/11486939/

18. Zametkin AJ, et al. Cerebral glucose metabolism in adults with hyperactivity of childhood onset. http://www.ncbi.nlm.nih.gov/pubmed/2233902
19. Chabot R J et al. Quantitative electroencephalographic profiles of children with attention deficit disorder. http://www.ncbi.nlm.nih.gov/sites/entrez/8915554
20. WHO news release. https://www.nih.gov/news-events/news-releases/brain-matures-few-years-late-adhd-follows-normal-pattern.
21. Krain L, et al. Brain development and ADHD. http://www.ncbi.nlm.nih.gov/pubmed/16480802
22. Winsberg B G, et al. Association of the dopamine transporter gene (DAT1) with poor methylphenidate response. http://www.ncbi.nlm.nih.gov/sites/entrez/10596245
23. Sheen VL, et al. Methylphenidate and continuous spike and wave during sleep in a child with attention deficit hyperactivity disorder. https://pubmed.ncbi.nlm.nih.gov/23827428/
24. Tamijani SMS, et al. Thyroid hormones: Possible roles in epilepsy pathology. https://pubmed.ncbi.nlm.nih.gov/26362394/
25. Sawicka-Gutaj N. et al. Relationship between thyroid hormones and central nervous system metabolism in physiological and pathological conditions. https://pubmed.ncbi.nlm.nih.gov/35771431/
26. Weiss RE, et al. Behavioral effects of liothyronine (L-T3) in children with attention deficit hyperactivity disorder in the presence and absence of resistance to thyroid. https://pubmed.ncbi.nlm.nih.gov/9226208/
27. Zwi M, et al. Parent training interventions for attention deficit hyperactivity disorder (ADHD) in children aged 5 to 18 years. https://pubmed.ncbi.nlm.nih.gov/22161373/
28. Greeley GH Jr, et al. Decreased serum 3,5,3'-triiodothyronine and thyroxine levels accompanying acute and chronic Ritalin treatment of developing rats. https://pubmed.ncbi.nlm.nih.gov/6766387/
29. Saper CB, et al. Hypothalamic regulation of sleep and circadian rhythms. Nature. 437 (7063): 1257–1263. doi:10.1038/nature04284.

Chapter 12: How can you identify ADHD in adults

1. Weiss MD. A guide to the treatment of adults with ADHD. https://www.webmd.com/add-adhd/long-term-risks-adhd-medications.

List of Common Complaints

Fatigue or Excessive Tiredness
- Obesity
- Cold extremities
- Loss of stamina
- Low morning temperature
- Slow recovery from disease
- Dry skin
- Dark circles under eyes

Circulatory System
- High cholesterol
- Heart disease
- High blood pressure
- High glucose

Gastrointestinal System
- Constipation
- Excessive gas
- Bad breath
- Stomach reflux
- Gastrointestinal
- Irritable bowel syndrome (IBS)
- *H pylori* infection
- *H pylori* infection (gastric cancer)
- Anal fissure
- Hemorrhoids

Respiratory System
- Asthma
- Any autoimmune disease
- Multiple sclerosis
- Cancer

Nervous System
- Carpal tunnel syndrome
- Generalized muscle spasms and pains
- Epilepsy
- Mental disease
- Low concentration
- Panic attacks
- ADD/ADHD
- Postpartum depression
- Depression
- Nervousness and anxiety

Disturbances in Females
- Irregular, longer, lighter,
  or heavier menstrual cycles
- PMS
- Infertility
- Miscarriage
- Severe menstrual cramps
- Myoma
- Loss of libido
- Leg cramps

Disturbances in Males
- Heart failure
- Gynecomastia
- Baldness
- Erectile dysfunction
- loss of libido
- Infertility
- Enlarged prostate

Inability to Lose Weight
- Swollen neck or goiter
- Afternoon energy crash
- Face edema
- Trembling, jittery
- Inability to exercise

Skin Diseases
- Loss of eyebrow hair (outer portion)
- Slow/Weak pulse (under 60 bpm)
- Atrial fibrillation attacks
- Heart palpitations

Food Allergies and Sensitivities
Gastrointestinal Disturbance
- Irritable bowel syndrome (IBS)
- *H pylori* infection
- *H pylori* infection (gastric cancer)
- Anal fissure
- Hemorrhoids
- Craving sweets
- Craving salt
- Liver/Gallbladder stones

Made in the USA
Coppell, TX
11 August 2024